Brain Stem Electric Response Audiometry

Michael E. Glasscock III, M.D., F.A.C.S.
C. Gary Jackson, M.D.
Anne Forrest Josey, M.S., C.C.C.A.

All of The Otology Group
Nashville, Tennessee

Associate Editor
Jerry L. Northern, Ph.D.

University of Colorado
Health Sciences Center
Denver, Colorado

1981

Thieme-Stratton, Inc. • New York
Georg Thieme Verlag • Stuttgart • New York

Publisher: Thieme-Stratton Inc.
           381 Park Avenue South
           New York, New York 10016

Brain Stem Electric Response Audiometry   ISBN 913258-93-8

Last digit is print number 9 8 7 6 5 4 3 2

PREFACE

This book is not meant to be a treatise on brain stem electric response audiometry (BERA), nor is it a reference work. It was written as a practical introduction to the clinical use of BERA for audiology students, residents, and practicing otolaryngologists. The Ph.D. audiologist with prior knowledge of BERA will not find this book intellectually stimulating.

We have attempted to standardize terminology as much as possible. This has been difficult to accomplish because the field is new and constantly changing. In some instances we have decided upon a term even though we realize that within a few months it might change. A prime example is the book's title, *Brain Stem Electric Response Audiometry*. Terminology for this procedure has shifted back and forth for the past two to three years. At present there is a move to use "Auditory Evoked Response Audiometry" which doubtless will spawn a new acronym, AERA. Although parts of this book may be dated by the time of publication, our intention is to provide an introduction to the subject as it relates to clinical practice. In this light, the book should serve its purpose for several years.

A section of test equipment was purposely omitted owing to the constant evolution of new equipment rendering each piece of hardware obsolete within two to three years of its manufacture. The underlying principles of neurophysiology and test methodology are less changeable, so that if one masters the test procedure on today's equipment, the knowledge can be easily transferred to the more sophisticated units of the future.

Above all, this book is clinically oriented, having been written with the clinical audiologist and the practicing otolaryngologist in mind. Its two sections deal with basic considerations (Chapters 1, 2, and 3) with clinical applications (Chapters 4 and 5). This arrangement should allow the individual to select an entry point for reading based upon his prior knowledge of BERA and what he wishes to obtain from the book.

This is not a cookbook on how to do BERA; the reader will not become proficient in performing and interpreting BERA tracings from this book. Rather, those who survive a reading of the book should have a solid working knowledge of BERA and its clinical applications. For technical proficiency in administering BERA, enrollment in one of the basic courses offered through the year is necessary.

CONTENTS

Brain Stem
Electric Response
Audiometry

Chapter One

AN INTRODUCTION TO BRAIN STEM ELECTRIC RESPONSE AUDIOMETRY

HISTORY

As brain stem electric response audiometry (BERA) assumes its position as an important diagnostic procedure, it is appropriate to review the major events leading to its widespread use in clinical audiometry. A glossary of pertinent terms and classifications follows our historical account. Our review is intended only as a preface to the clinical chapters of this book. The reader is referred elsewhere for more detail.[1-4]

The origins of BERA can be traced to the animal experiments of the 19th century. In 1875, Caton[5] first reported that there was electrical activity in the brain, which could be demonstrated by evoked potentials in the rabbit. He was also the first to notice the unexpected spontaneous ossilations of the baseline that were later to become known as the electrocorticogram.

Danilevsky[6] working in Russia, studied the spontaneous electrical activity of the brain in dogs in or around 1877. Essentially, he rediscovered evoked potentials in the dog rather than in the rabbit. Unlike Caton, he was aware of the auditory potentials. Between 1883 and 1891 Fleischl von Marxow,[7] Beck,[8] and Gotch and Horsley[9] actively pursued the recording of electrical activity of the brain in a variety of experimental animals, but it was Pravdich-Neminsky[10] in 1913 who first photographed the record of an animal electroencephalogram with a string galvanometer.

Until more sophisticated equipment was designed, researchers were limited in their range of activity. In the early part of the 20th century, electrophysiologists were working under very primitive conditions owing to the lack of sophisticated equipment. It was not until 1920 that an electrical amplifier was used in a physiological experiment by Forbes and Thacher;[11] the cathode-ray oscilloscope was not in general use until 1922. In the 1930s, oscilloscopic images were made bright enough and electrical amplifiers were stable enough to allow neurophysiologists to devote their time to experiments rather than to equipment problems.

In 1927, Forbes, Miller, and O'Connor[12] presented a series of rapidly repeated clicks to a cat's ear and were able to record the volley of nerve impulses. Wever and Bray[13] performed a series of experiments that led to the development of the cochlear microphonic 2 years later by Saul and Davis.[14] Wever and his associate listened to words spoken into a cat's ear that had been recorded and fed into a telephone receiver. To their amazement, the words were intelligible!

By 1935, Derbyshire and Davis[15] had established the hair cells of the organ of Corti as the generator of the cochlear microphonic. Their work was published as a definitive study of the action potentials in the auditory nerve. Four years later a microintracellular electrode was developed by Hodgkin and Huxley[16] to record the membrane potential and the action potential of the giant axon of the squid. In 1943, Galambos and Davis[17] reported the first response areas and characteristic frequencies of auditory units in the cat. Tasaki[18] was responsible for penetrating the first-order fibers of the cochlear nerve in the guinea pig. Kiang,[19] by use of micromanipulators and computers, obtained discharge patterns in single fibers in the cat auditory nerve in 1965.

By the early 1960s, neurophysiologists were beginning to record evoked auditory potentials. The groundwork for their studies had been laid by the early investigators of the human electroencephalogram (EEG). The alpha rhythm was first demonstrated by Berger[20] in 1929. Loomis (as referenced in Davis)[4] working independently, rediscovered the EEG and was responsible for naming the ''K'' complex in 1935. By 1954, Dawson[21] was able to use the first electronic response averager, an analogue device with 124 time points and a mechanical revolving commutator to charge each condenser in turn. The response averager was employed in the recording of the slow somatosensory cortical responses to electrical stimulation of the ulna nerve in the human. By 1961, Davis[24] had acquired a digital computer and began using it extensively in his electrophysiology experiments.

Subsequently, in 1963 the New York Academy of Arts and Sciences sponsored a symposium that brought together investigators in the various fields of averaged potentials, including visual, somatosensory, auditory, myogenic, and neurogenic. The following year a program was presented in Toronto concerning the identification and management of the young deaf child by use of electric response audiometry. Because of the widening interest and expanding knowledge of the subject of evoked potentials, the International Electric Response Audiometry Study Group was founded in 1968.

By 1968, slow cortical response audiometry under sedation was being attempted in some centers; however, it proved to be unreliable in a clinical setting and never gained widespread acceptance. At the same time, Yoshie and associates,[22] Aran and LeBert,[23] and Sohmer and Feinmesser[24] applied the technique of response averaging to the ear and introduced electrocochleography (E Coch G). Because of the need to place an electrode directly on the basal coil of the cochlea, this procedure never gained wide acceptance in the United States. Sohmer and Feinmesser were able to use "far field" electrodes to perform E Coch G by placing the active electrode in the ear canal rather than through the tympanic membrane and on to the cochlea. By 1971, Jewett and Williston[25] had established a definitive description of BERA, and in 1974 Hecox and Galambos[26] expanded this definition to the audiometry of infants and adults. From 1974 to the present time there have been numerous contributors to the clinical use of BERA. Starr and Hamilton[27] are renowned for their description of the possible origins of waves I through V and for having demonstrated the value of BERA in the diagnosis of central nervous system disease. Selters and Brackmann,[28] as well as House and Brackmann[31] and Glasscock and associates,[30] have shown that BERA is highly reliable in the demonstration of cerebellopontine angle lesions such as acoustic tumors.

With the widespread use of BERA in a clinical setting, equipment manufacturers have made a concerted effort to simplify and modernize their products. Throughout the country, courses in the practical use of BERA are presented, and there is little question that this diagnostic procedure has established for itself a permanent position in the modern evaluation scheme of the auditory system. The cumbersome, experimental recording of evoked auditory potentials has moved from the laboratory into the audiology clinic, where it is now a practical diagnostic study.

GLOSSARY

Classification of Auditory Evoked Potentials

Of the many different electrical responses to auditory stimuli, most arise in the central nervous system, some are generated in the cochlea, and still others are reflex responses in muscles. In order to discuss BERA it is important to understand the nomenclature. Therefore, the following terms set forth by the London Symposium of the International Electric Response Audiometry Study Group (1975) are presented.

Evoked Potentials and Electric Responses

By definition a response is evoked. Thus, "evoked response" is somewhat redundant. Potentials are evoked; therefore, evoked potential and electrical response are proper designations.

V (Vertex) Potentials

On the basis of electrode placement, the first distinction among evoked potentials is anatomical, "at the vertex" or "in the ear." In the first subdivision, one or two reference electrodes are placed on the ear lobe or mastoid while the active electrode is attached to the top of the head or vertex. Vertex potentials measured in this fashion are classified by latency as fast, middle, slow, or late. This method of recording evoked potentials is called "far field" technique.

The second subdivision is referred to as E Coch G, and the reference electrodes are placed on the ear lobe and the active electrode is placed within the middle ear or external auditory canal. If classified by latency (as the V potentials), these evoked potentials would be referred to as the first potentials.

Continuing Response

The second distinction among evoked potentials is physiological and is based upon whether it is a continuing (alternating current [AC]) or sustained (direct current [DC]) potential. The continuing potentials have been assigned specific names and abbreviations.

Cochlear Microphonic (CM). A continuing AC response generated chiefly by the external hair cells in the organ of Corti.

Summating Potential (SP). A continuing DC response generated in both internal and external hair systems, depending upon whether it is negative or positive.

Frequency Following Response (FFR). A continuing AC response generated in several nuclei of the brain stem.

Sustained Cortical Potential (SCP). A continuing DC response generated in the cerebral (auditory) cortex.

Contingent Negative Variant (CNV). A very late DC shift developing in certain situations between a warning signal and an expected imperative stimulus.

On-effects

The on-effects are subdivided on the basis of their latencies as to fast, middle, slow, or late. A particular wave is designated by P if it is vertex-positive and by N if it is vertex-negative. A subscript is used to give the on-effects', most characteristic latency in a normal hearing adult at a sensation level of 60 decibels (dB). For example, a late cortex wave would be P_{300}.

REFERENCES

1. Brazier, M. A. B.: The historical development of neurophysiology, in Field, J., Magoun, H. W., Hall, V. E. (eds.): *Handbooks of Physiology, Section 1: Neurophysiology.* Washinton, D.C., American Physiological Society, 1959, vol. 1, chap. 1.
2. Brazier, M. A. B.: *A History of the Electrical Activity of the Brain,* New York, The MacMillan Co., 1961.
3. Neff, W. D. and Keidel, W. D. (eds.): *Handbook of Sensory Physiology.* Berlin, Heidelberg, New York, Springer-Verlag, 1974, vol V/2.
4. Davis, H.: Principles of electric response audiometry, Ann Otol Rhinol Laryngol 85(Suppl 28): 1976.
5. Caton, R.: The electric currents of the brain. Br Med J 2:278, 1875.
6. Danilevsky, V. Y.: Investigations into the physiology of the brain. Thesis, University of Karkov, 1877.
7. Fleischl von Marxow, E.: Mittheilung betreffend die Physiologie der Hirnrinde. Zbl Physiol 4:538, 1890.
8. Beck, A.: Die Bestimmung der Localisation der Gehirn—und Rückenmarkfunctionen vermittelst der electrischen Erscheinungen. Cbl Physiol 4:473-476, 1890.
9. Gotch, F., and Horsley, V.: Über den Gebrauch der Elektricität für die Lokalisierung der Erregungsercheinungen im Centralnervensystem. Zbl Physiol 4:649-651, 1891.
10. Pravdich-Neminsky, V. V.: Ein Versuch der Registrierung der elektrischen Gehirnerscheinungen. Zbl Physiol 27:951-960, 1913.
11. Forbes, A., and Thacher, C.: Amplification of action currents with the electron tube in recording with the string galvanometer. Am J Physiol 52:409-471, 1920.
12. Forbes, A., Miller, R. H., O'Connor, J.: Electric responses to acoustic stimuli in the decerebrate animal. Am J Physiol 80:363-380, 1927.
13. Wever, E. G., and Bray, C. W.: The nature of acoustic response: the relation between sound frequency and frequency of impulses in the auditory nerve. J Exp Psychol 13:373-387, 1930.
14. Saul, L. J., and Davis, H.: Action currents in the central nervous system: I. Action currents of the auditory tracts. Arch New Psychiatr 28:1104-1116, 1932.
15. Derbyshire, A. J., and Davis, H.: The action potentials of the auditory nerve. Am J Physiol 113:476-504, 1935.
16. Hodgkin, A. L., and Huxley, A. F.: Action potentials recorded from inside a nerve fiber. Nature 144:710-711, 1939.
17. Galambos, R., and Davis, H.: The response of single auditory-nerve fibers to acoustic stimulation. J Neurophysiol 6:39-57, 1943.
18. Tasaki, I: Nerve impulses in individual auditory nerve fibers of guinea pig. J Neurophysiol 17:97-122, 1954.
19. Kiang, NY-S: *Discharge Patterns of Single Fiber in the Cat's Auditory Nerve.* Cambridge, MIT Press, 1965.
20. Berger, H.: Uber das Elektrenkephalogramm des Menschen. I. Arch f Psychiatr 87:527-570, 1929.
21. Dawson, G. D.: A summation technique for the detection of small evoked potentials. Electroencephalogr Clin Neurophysiol 6:65-84, 1954.
22. Yoshie N., Ohashi, T., and Suzuki, T.: Nonsurgical recording of auditory nerve action potentials in man. Laryngoscope 77:76-85, 1967.
23. Aran, J. M., and LeBert, G.: Les responses nerveuses cochleaeres chez l'homme, image du fonctionnement de l'oreille et nouveau test d'audiometrie objective. Rev Laryngol Otol Rhinol (Bord) 89:361-378, 1968.
24. Sohmer, H., and Feinmesser, M.: Cochlear action potentials recorded from the external ear in man. Ann Otol Rhinol Laryngol 76:427-435, 1967.
25. Jewett, D. L., and Williston, J. S.: Auditory evoked far-fields averaged from the scalp of humans. Brain 94:681-696, 1971.
26. Hecox, K., and Galambos, R.: Brain stem auditory evoked responses in human infants and adults. Arch Otolaryngol 99:30-33, 1974.

27. Starr, A., and Hamilton, A.: Correlation between confirmed sites of neurological lesions of far-field auditory brain stem responses. Electroencephalogr Clin Neurophysiol 41:595–608, 1976.

28. Selters, W. A., and Brackmann, D. E.: Acoustic tumor detection with brain stem electric response audiometry. Arch Otolaryngol 103:181–187, 1977.

29. House, J. W., and Brackmann, D. E., Brain stem audiometry in neurotologic diagnosis. Arch Otolaryngol 105:305, 1979.

30. Glassock, M. E., Jackson, C. G., Josey, A. F., Dickins, J. R., and Wiet, R. J.: Brain stem evoked response audiometry in a clinical practice. Laryngoscope 89:1021–1034, 1979.

Chapter Two

THE AUDITORY SYSTEM

This chapter provides a synopsis of the anatomy and physiology of the auditory system as a basis for our discussion of brain stem electric response audiometry (BERA) methodology and clinical application. The reader is referred to the following publications for more detail: the anatomy of the outer, middle, and inner ear is particularly well covered in *Gray's Anatomy*,[1] the detailed structure of the cochlea and the central pathways of the auditory system can be found in Schuknecht's *Pathology of the Ear*,[2] and the physiology of the auditory system has been described extensively by Davis.[3]

ANATOMY OF THE AUDITORY SYSTEM

The auditory system consists of the outer, middle, and inner ear, the cochlear nerve, the cochlear nuclei, the brain stem pathways, and the auditory cortex.

The Outer Ear

The outer ear consists of the auricle (pinna) and the external auditory canal. The auricle is an ovoid structure, with its larger portion located superiorly. The lateral surface is concave, having numerous depressions and protrusions, each assigned a specific name. The auricle consists of one large piece of cartilage covered by thin skin closely adherent to the cartilage and continuous with the epithelium of the external auditory meatus. The vascular supply is from the posterior branch of the external carotid artery, the superficial temporal artery, and the occipital artery.

The sensory nerves are the great auricular (cervical plexus), the auricular branch of the vagus, the auriculotemporal branch of the mandibular (V-3), and the lesser occipital (cervical plexus) (Fig. 2–1).

The external canal is two-thirds bone and one-third cartilage. The skin is thin and closely adherent to the underlying structures. The overall length is approximately 2.5 centimeters (cm), with the cerumen glands located in

11

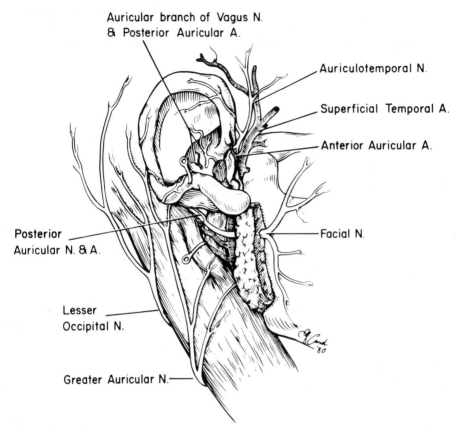

Auricular branch of Vagus N.
& Posterior Auricular A.

Auriculotemporal N.

Superficial Temporal A.

Anterior Auricular A.

Posterior
Auricular N. & A.

Facial N.

Lesser
Occipital N.

Greater Auricular N.

Figure 2-1. The sensory nerves are the great auricular (cervical plexus), auricular branch of the vagus, auriculotemporal branch of the mandibular (V-3), and the lesser occipital (cervical plexus).

the outer one-third of the canal and placed superiorly. The junction of the cartilaginous and bony canals is referred to as the isthmus. The cartilage of the canal is deficient anteriorly, where two-thirds of the fissures are present. The bony canal is narrower than the cartilaginous portion and terminates medially at the tympanic sulcus. This V-shaped or grooved portion receives the fibrous annulus of the tympanic membrane. The sulcus is deficient superiorly in the area known as the notch of Rivinus.

Anterior to the bony canal lies the temporomandibular joint, and posterior to it are the mastoid air cells. The arteries supplying the external canal derive from the posterior auricular, internal maxillary, and the temporal arteries. The external canal is innervated by the auriculotemporal branch of the mandibular nerve (V-3) and the auricular branch of the vagus.

The Middle Ear

The middle ear comprises the tympanic cavity, the eustachian tube, the tympanic membrane, and the ossicles.

Tympanic Membrane

The tympanic membrane closes the medial end of the external auditory canal. It has three distinct layers. The middle layer consists of interlacing collagenous fibers radiating away from the handle of the malleus (first ossicle) and the circumference of the membrane form a thick ring (fibrous anulus) that rests in the tympanic sulcus of the bony external auditory canal. The outer surface of this fibrous middle layer is covered by skin that is continuous with the ear canal, but that does not contain rete pegs. The inner surface of the fibrous layer is covered with a mucous membrane that is continuous with that of the middle ear (Fig. 2-2).

The tympanic membrane is semitransparent, and the portion containing the fibrous layer is referred to as the pars tensa. A small triangular area of the drum lying superior to the short process of the malleus is known as the pars flacida or Schrapnell's membrane. Two fibrous folds extending

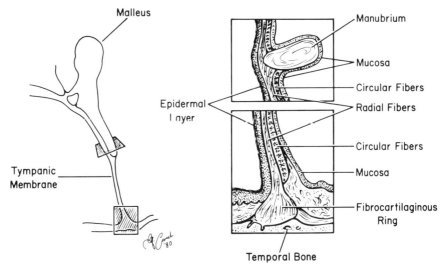

Figure 2-2. The tympanic membrane closes the medial end of the external auditory canal. It has three distinct layers. The middle layer consists of interlacing collagenous fibers radiating away from the handle of the malleus (first ossicle), and the circumference of the membrane forms a thick ring (fibrous annulus) that rests in the tympanic sulcus of the bony external auditory canal. The outer surface of this fibrous middle layer is covered by skin which is continuous with the ear canal, but which does not contain Redepegs. The inner surface of the fibrous layer is covered with mucous membrane which is continuous with that of the middle ear.

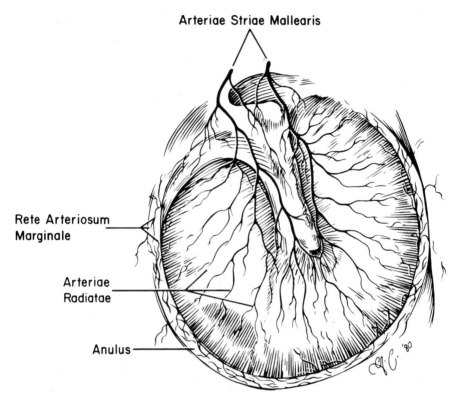

Figure 2-3. The main vascular supply enters the tympanic membrane superiorly and is derived from the internal maxillary artery. Additional vascularity comes from the postauricular and tympanic arteries.

from the malleus to the edge of the notch of Rivinus are the anterior and posterior malleolar ligaments.

The tympanic membrane is cone-shaped, the most depressed part of the concavity or umbo corresponding to the tip of the handle of the malleus.

The main vascular supply enters the tympanic membrane superiorly and is derived from the internal maxillary artery. Additional vascularity comes from the postauricular and tympanic arteries (Fig. 2–3).

The eardrum is innervated by the auriculotemporal branch of the mandibular nerve, the auricular branch of the vagus nerve, and the tympanic branch of the glossopharyngeal nerve.

Tympanic Cavity

The middle ear or tympanic cavity is an irregular air-filled space lying within the temporal bone. The area just medial to the tympanic membrane is the tympanic cavity, whereas the space above the membrane is the epitympanic recess or attic. This space contains the head of the malleau and the body of the incus. Measuring from the attic to the floor of the middle ear cavity (hypotympanicum) and from the anterior to the posterior, the space is approximately 15 × 15 millimeters (mm). The transverse diameter measures 6 mm in the attic and 4 mm in the hypotympanicum. Just medial to the umbo, the space is only 2-mm wide (Fig. 2–4).

The roof of the tympanic cavity is called the tegmen tympani and consists of the thin layer of bone separating the attic from the dura overlying the temporal lobe. The floor or hypotympanicum consists of air cells similar to those found in the mastoid. The inferior aspect of this cell system consists of a thin layer of bone separating it from the dome of the jugular bulb. Posteriorly, the tympanic cavity communicates with the antrum of the mastoid and anteriorly with the eustachian or auditory tube,

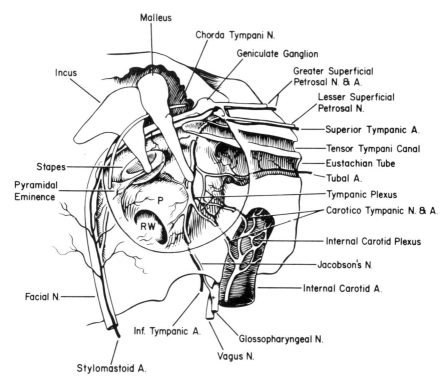

Figure 2–4. The middle ear or tympanic cavity is an irregular air-filled space lying within the temporal bone. The area just medial to the tympanic membrane is the tympanic cavity. The space above the membrane is the epitympanic recess or attic. This space contains the head of the malleus and body of the incus. Measuring from the attic to the floor of the middle ear cavity (hypotympanicum) and from anterior to posterior, the space is approximately 15 × 15 mm. The transverse diameter measures 6 mm in the attic and 4 mm in the hypotympanicum. Just medial to the umbo, the space is only 2 mm wide.

which connects the cavity to the nasopharynx. The bony portion is approximately one-third its length, the remaining two-thirds being cartilaginous. The bony cartilaginous junction is known as the isthmus. As the tube enters the nasopharynx, there is an elevation of cartilage just posterior to the orifice called the torus tabaris. Behind this structure is a depression referred to as Rosenmüller's fossa. The mucous membrane of the middle ear cavity and the eustachian tube is respiratory in nature and contains cilia.

Just inferior to the eustachian tube and anterior to the lower half of the tympanic cavity lies the carotid canal containing the internal carotid artery.

The medial wall of the middle ear space comprises the basal coil of the cochlea (auditory portion of the inner ear) and is known as the promontory.

The fenestra vestibuli (oval window) opens into the vestibule of the inner ear. Its greatest diameter is in the horizontal plane. The third ossicle (stapes) lies in the oal window.

The fenestra cochlea (round window) lies below and behind the oval windows and communicates with the scala tympani of the cochlea. It is closed by a three-layered secondary membrane (round window membrane) separating the fluid-filled scala tympani of the cochlea from the middle ear cavity.

The semicanal of the tensor tympani muscle, as well as the horizontal or middle ear segment of the facial nerve canal, are prominent projections from the medial wall into the cavity. The second middle ear muscle, the stapedius, protrudes from the pyramidal eminence, where it attaches to the neck of the stapes.

Ossicles

The ossicles themselves are known as the malleus, incus, and stapes. The malleus has a head, neck, short or lateral process, and a handle that is buried within the fibrous layer of the tympanic membrane. The incus has a body, long and short processes, and an articular surface that interlocks with the head of the malleus. The lenticular process of the incus is a small, cartilaginous structure connecting the long process of the incus to the head of the stapes. The stapes itself looks like the stirrup of an English saddle. The footplate lies in the oval window and is held in place by a fibrous ring, the anular ligament. Two crura or arches extend from the anterior and posterior portions of the footplate, forming the neck. The capitulum or head of the stapes rests on the neck and is covered by cartilage. The malleus and incus are suspended in the attic by ligaments that allow them to vibrate as a unit.

The facial nerve passes through the middle ear and mastoid in the fallopian canal. In its mastoid segment, the facial nerve gives off the chorda tympani nerve, which transverses the tympanic cavity and exits through the iter chordae anterius and the petrotympanic fissure to supply taste to the anterior two-thirds of the tongue.

Vascular supply of the tympanic cavity is by way of the inferior tympanic artery, which is a branch of the ascending pharyngeal artery from the external carotid artery. The caroticotympanic branches from the internal carotid artery, the stylomastoid branch of the postauricular artery, and the tympanic branch of the internal maxillary artery also contribute to the vascular supply of the tympanic cavity.

The tympanic branch of the glossopharyngeal nerve (Jacobson's nerve) enters the tympanic cavity in the hypotympanum, courses across the promontory, and exits just medial to the cochleariformis process. It then enters the middle fossa as the lesser superficial petrosal nerve and exits through a fissure or foramen of its own, terminating in the otic ganglion.

The Inner Ear

The inner ear consists of three semicircular canals, the vestibule, and the cochlea (Fig. 2–5). The bone or labyrinth of the inner ear is compact and very dense. The labyrinth is suspended in a lattice work of air cells within the apex of the temporal bone. Inside this bony structure is a membranous labyrinth.

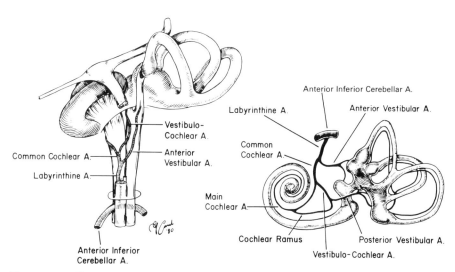

Figure 2-5. The inner ear consists of the three semicircular canals, the vestibule, and the cochlea.

Semicircular Canals. Since this discussion is primarily concerned with the auditory system, the vestibular apparatus will not be discussed in detail. There are three semicircular canals: the horizontal or lateral, the posterior, and the superior. These canals open into the vestibule, the superior and posterior canals having a common crus. Thus, there are three semicircular canals with five openings into the vestibule. Each canal contains a corresponding membranous counterpart. There is an ampulated or swollen end of each canal containing the neuroepithelium of the peripheral vestibular system.

Vestibule

The vestibule is the central part of the osseous labyrinth lying between the semicircular canals and the cochlea. Its medial wall has two depressions, the recessus ellipticus, which holds the membranous utricle, and the recessus sphericus, in which the saccule rests. Running parallel to the common crus is the opening for the vestibular aqueduct. The medial wall is perforated allowing the fibers of the vestibular nerve to enter the utricle, the saccule, and the superior and horizontal ampulae.

Cochlea

The cochlea is the peripheral center for hearing and is an extremely complicated structure. Its bony contours resemble a common snail shell, as its coil makes approximately two and two-thirds turns. Measuring about 5 mm from base to apex and 9 mm across its base, the cochlea contains a conical-shaped central axis known as the modiolus, from which projects a delicate ledge of bone—the osseous spiral lamina. Extending from the spiral lamina is the basilar membrane separating the cochlea into two chambers that communicate with each other at the apex of the modiolus by a small opening—the helicotrema.

The modiolus is the central conical core of the cochlea, wide at the base and narrow at the apex. The bony canal of the cochlea is about 30 mm in length and approximately 3 mm in diameter and communicates through three openings to other structures: The round window (fenestra rotundum) is closed by the round window membrane; the second opening connects the cochlea to the vestibule; and the cochlear aqueduct communicates with the subarachnoid space. The latter structure transmits cerebrospinal fluid from the subarachnoid space into the scala tympani of the cochlea.

The cochlea is divided into three separate chambers by the osseous lamina, the basilar membrane, and Reissner's membrane (Fig. 2-6). The chambers are the scala media (cochlear duct), the scala vestibuli, and the scala tympani. The scala media is formed by the basilar and Reissner's

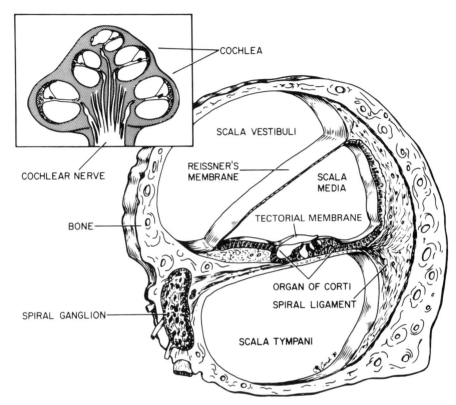

Figure 2-6. The cochlea is divided into three separate chambers by the osseous lamina, the basilar membrane, and Reissner's membrane.

membranes and contains the organ of Corti, which sits on the inner part of the basilar membrane. The organ of Corti consists of epithelial elements forming two rows of rod-like bodies known as the inner and outer rods or pillars of Corti. The bases of the pillars are supported on the basilar membrane, and the tops incline toward each other to form an arch or tunnel of Corti. The inner row of rods contain the inner hair cells (single), whereas the outer side of the rods support three or four rows of similar cells, termed the supporting cells of Dieters and Hensen. The free ends of the outer hair cells are embedded in the tectorial membrane. The inner hair cells number about 3500 and the outer hair cells number about 12,000.

Along the outer aspect of the scala media lies the stria vascularis, a vascular meshwork of arteries, which is thought to produce endolymph, the clear fluid found throughout the membranous labyrinth. The scala vestibuli and tympani, bony vestibule, and bony semicircular canals contain a clear fluid, perilymph, which is thought to arise from the cerebrospinal fluid through the cochlear aqueduct. Perilymph and endolymph are similar in nature, but endolymph is high in potassium ion concentration and perilymph is high in sodium ion concentration.

The Auditory Nerve

The staticoacoustic nerve (cranial nerve VIII) comprises the vestibular nerve (superior and inferior divisions and Scarpa's ganglion) and the cochlear nerve. The number of myelinated nerve fibers in the cochlear nerve of humans averages around 35,000. There are two types of cochlear afferent neurons. Type I neurons, which account for 95 per cent of the total, have large cell bodies and are connected exclusively to the inner hair cells. Type II neurons, which constitute the remaining 5 per cent, innervate the outer hair cells and do not have myelinated sheaths. Each interval hair cell is innervated by ten Type II neurons. The nerve cells are located in the spiral ganglion within the modiolus and the osseous spiral lamina. Axons pass by way of the cochlear nerve through the modiolus and internal auditory canal and across the cerebellopontine angle with the facial nerve (cranial nerve VII) to enter the brain stem. There is an orderly spatial arrangement of the cochlear neurons as they pass through the cochlear nerve to the brain stem nuclei. Fibers from the basal turn are located in the peripheral and inferior portions of the nerve trunk, and apical fibers are situated in the central region.

Central Auditory Pathways

Within the brain stem each fiber of the cochlear nerve divides into an anterior branch terminating in the anterior part of the ventral cochlear nucleus, and into a longer posterior branch that divides again, one fiber entering the posterior part of the ventral cochlear nucleus, and the other investing the dorsal cochlear nucleus. Thus, the major afferent input is into the ventral nucleus. The cells of the dorsal cochlear nucleus send their axons across the midline, where they ascend in the medial division of the contralateral lateral lemniscus. The ascending axons from the dorsal nucleus terminate in the dorsal nucleus of the lateral lemniscus and in the inferior colliculus.

The cell bodies from the ventral cochlear nucleus distribute axons to the ipsilateral and contralateral superior olivary complex, where they ascend the lateral lemniscus to terminate in its nucleus and the inferior colliculus.

The distal projections from the inferior colliculus are primarily to the

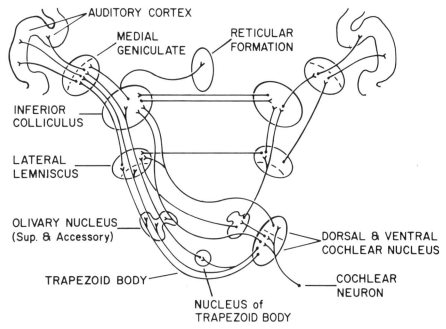

Figure 2-7. The distal projections from the inferior colliculus are primarily to the medial geniculate body and thence to the auditory cortex in the temporal lobe of the brain.

medial geniculate body and thence to the auditory cortex in the temporal lobe of the brain (Fig. 2-7).

There are synaptic connections between the dorsal nucleus of the lateral lemniscus and the inferior colliculus. In lower primates[4] as the auditory fibers ascend from the cochlea to the cortex, there is a progressively larger population of neurons with the cortex containing some 10,200,000 neurons.

Rasmussen[5] described a population of descending or efferent neurons that parallel the ascending pathways and link the auditory cortex with the lower auditory centers and the organ of Corti. These fibers are referred to as the olivocochlear bundle. The exact nature of their function is not known.

PHYSIOLOGY OF THE AUDITORY SYSTEM

The function of the auditory system is dependent upon three factors: (1) The structural composition of the outer, middle, and inner ear; (2) the production of electrical impulses originating in the cochlea; and (3) the transmission of these impulses through the cochlear nerve and the central neural pathways.

The Mechanism of Hearing

The auricle is of little auditory significance in the human. Its location on either side of the head provides an acoustic baffle between the two ears in order to assure that the direction of sound can be detected. In humans the whole head is used to scan for sound as opposed to the individual scanning ability of the auricle in lower animal forms. Sound is created by vibrations of air particles, which are collected by the auricle and external canal and are then transmitted to the tympanic membrane. The chief function of the middle ear is to provide an impedance match between the air of the external auditory canal and the fluid of the cochlea, thereby efficiently delivering acoustical energy to the organ of Corti.

The external auditory canal has a resonant frequency of 4000 Hertz (Hz), which accounts for an increase of sensitivity of about 10 dB at this frequency. The middle ear has a resonant frequency of approximately 1700 Hz. Therefore, combined with the external canal, the overall acoustic frequency response of the ear is 800 to 6000 Hz.

The vibrating air particles set the tympanic membrane into motion, which, in turn, drives the ossicular chain. The large surface area of the tympanic membrane—80 mm²—compared to the small area of the stapes footplate—3 mm²—creates a hydraulic effect in a 20:1 ratio, which allows the weak air vibrations to set the perilymph of the vestibule into motion.

As the stapes moves into the vestibule, a traveling wave is set up in the basilar membrane moving toward the scala tympani. The round window membrane bulges outward to compensate for the inward motion of the stapes, since the fluid cannot be compressed. When the movement is slow, some fluid also flows through the helicotrema. The basilar membrane is narrow at the base and wide at the apex, so that high frequencies are detected in the base and low frequencies in the apex. Thus, the cochlea is a mechanical frequency analyzer. As the basilar membrane bulges in response to vibrations of the stapes footplate, the hair cells of the organ of Corti are bent by the movement of the tectoral membrane. Bending of the hair cells releases energy in the form of bioelectrical potentials, which are responsible for excitation of the auditory nerve fibers. The electrical activity is then transmitted by the cochlear nerve to the central pathways and by way of the brain stem to the auditory cortex, where integration takes place.

Electrical Responses of the Cochlea

The electrical activity of the central nervous system can be detected on the body surface and recorded thus making possible the science of electrocardiography (ECG) and electroencephalography (EEG). Similarly, the electrical impulses generated by the cochlea and central auditory pathways can be detected and recorded, making electrocochleography (E Coch G) and brain stem electric response audiometry (BERA) possible.

Action Potentials

If the electrical activity of the cochlea is synchronized into definite groups or volleys, as in response to clicks or successive sound waves of a low-frequency tone, the corresponding action potentials can be recorded by placing an electrode on the round window and one on the neck. Action potentials are recorded as the impulses pass through the modiolus just before they enter the internal auditory canal. Action potentials demonstrate an all-or-none "spike" response common to nerve fibers having a definite threshold followed by a refractory period.

Intracellular Potentials

With microelectrodes it is possible to measure the electrical potential within a single cell. The intracellular potential of the hair cells, nerve fibers, and supporting cells of the cochlea are negative and vary in strength from -80 to -20 millivolts (mv).

Endocochlear Potential

The endolymph in the scala media has a positive ($+80$ mv) electrical potential relative to the perilymph in the scalae tympani and vestibuli as well as to the perilymph in the spiral ligament and extracochlear tissues. The so-called endocochlear potential is dependent on an adequate supply of oxygen and falls rapidly in the anoxic experimental animal. The endocochlear potential is modified with displacement of the structures within the cochlea. As the basilar membrane moves toward the scala tympani and the stapes are driven into the oval window, there is a 5- to 10-mv increase in the positive potential. Outward movement of the stapes produces a reduction in the potential. Changes in the endocochlear potential are related to displacement rather than velocity and are sustained as long as the displacement occurs.

The source of the endocochlear potential is the stria vascularis. The changes in the potential that occur with displacement are generated in the organ of Corti (hair cells), but this organ is not responsible for the resting positive potential.

Cochlear Microphonic and Summating Potentials

Acoustical stimulation by the bending of cochlear hair cells produces a cochlear microphonic (CM) and two summating potentials (SP), both positive and negative. The CM is directly proportional to the displacement of the cochlear partition and therefore reproduces the wave form of the acoustical stimulus. The summating potentials reproduce the form of an envelope of the original acoustical signal. Both the CM and SP are linear and are related to the intensity of the acoustic stimulus; they do not exhibit a "threshold" like that of all-or-none action potentials. There is no evidence to suggest an all-or-none response in the hair cells or of a refractory period; therefore the CM and the SP demonstrate little or no fatigue or adaptation.

The CM is dependent upon oxygen as is the endocochlear potential, but is affected by certain injuries that leave the endocochlear potential intact.

The SP is observed on the oscilloscope as a displacement of the base line record on which the CM is superimposed. With toxic injury to the cochlea (anoxia, and so forth), the CM decreases and the negative SP increases. Likewise, a decrease in the positive potential is accompanied by an increase in the negative potential. The positive and negative potentials are thought to originate in the inner hair cell system, whereas the CM and the positive SP probably arise in the external hair cells.

The full sequence of changes depends upon the state of the cochlea, the position of the electrodes, and the frequency of the tone burst employed to produce the responses.

Volleys and Latencies

When the auditory nerve is stimulated with a single click, a sharp, well-synchronized volley of action potentials is produced. The initial response is referred to as N1. Apparently N1 and N2 result from repetitive firing of some, but not all, of the fibers owing to the refractory period of nerve fibers (Fig. 2–8).

The successive sound waves of a steady tone between 2000 and 4000 Hz give rise to similar, but smaller, volleys of action potentials that clearly reproduce the frequency of the tone, although no one fiber responds to every sound wave. At 1000 Hz or below, N1 is produced in the basal turn of the cochlea, in which the partition moves almost in phase as a unit. Different latencies of response account for less and less perfect synchronization of the impulses as frequency increases. Above 4000 Hz there is no synchronization either visible on the oscilloscope or audible. By using a high-frequency tone burst there is a well-synchronized N1 and N2 and sometimes N3. The latency of N1 shortens from 2 milliseconds (msec) near threshold to 1 msec as intensity increases. Latency is related to rise-time, intensity, and frequency of the acoustical signal.

Latency of action potentials is a reflection of the conduction time

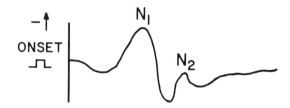

Figure 2-8. When the auditory nerve is stimulated with a single click, a sharp, well-synchronized volley of action potentials is produced. The initial response is referred to as N1. Apparently N1 and N2 result from repetitive firing of some, but not all, of the fibers owing to the refractory period of nerve fibers.

within the nonmedullated dendritic branches of the organ of Corti. As the volley passes through the modiolus it is recorded and measured from the beginning of the CM to the bottom of the action potential spike. There is no latency between the mechanical movement of the cochlear partition and the CM.

Below 3000 Hz, each sound wave acts more like an individual stimulus. Excitation occurs as the scalae media and vestibuli become more negative relative to the scala tympani, namely with outward movement of the stapes.

Single Fiber Activity

The single nerve fibers of the auditory system are 2.5 to 4.0 microns in diameter. If these fibers are probed with a microelectrode and the auditory system is stimulated with a brief tone burst, the resulting spike responses are similar to those from myelinated nerve fibers of similar size in other parts of the body. The auditory fibers give single or repetitive responses and will demonstrate either low or high thresholds. Most are selective with respect to frequency in that they demonstrate a sharp and stable cut-off frequency above which they fail to respond regardless of the intensity of the stimulation. Almost all fibers have cut-offs above 1000 Hz, but some have cut-offs as low as 100 Hz.

The phenomenon of adaptation is explained on the basis of a gradually diminishing rate of irregular discharges that continue after presenting a continuing tonal stimulation to the auditory nerve.

As the stimulus increases, N1 increases along a sigmoid curve before reaching a plateau and once again rising much more rapidly. The tendency of single nerve fibers to group into high-threshold and low-threshold classes explains the nonlinear behavior of N1 in the whole-nerve response.

Efferent Inhibitory Action

The efferent auditory pathway consists of fibers extending from the cortex to the cochlea. Stimulation of the olivocochlear tract (bundle of

Rasmussen) in the medulla has an inhibitory effect on the action potential response to clicks. N1 is reduced, but the CM is unaltered. The purpose of this efferent pathway is not understood.

PATHOPHYSIOLOGY OF THE AUDITORY SYSTEM

The normal transmission of sound waves through the middle ear, cochlea, and central pathways to the cerebral cortex presumes on a functioning auditory system. Pathological changes can occur at any point in the mechanism, resulting in hearing loss or disruption of the orderly transfer of neural impulses through the brain stem pathways, which is referred to as dysynchrony.

Hearing Loss

There are three basic types of hearing loss: conductive, sensorineural, or a combination of the two, which is referred to as mixed loss.

Conductive Hearing Loss

Conductive losses are caused by blockage of sound vibrations in their transfer through the external auditory canal and middle ear. The simplest and one of the commonest forms of conductive hearing loss results from an accumulation of excessive cerumen in the external auditory canal (Fig. 2-9). The resulting hearing loss can reach 60 dB air conduction levels with impaction. Happily, this type of loss is easily reversible by removing the cerumen. A foreign body occluding the external canal is not an unusual finding. Children push pencils, erasers, beans, and all manner of small objects into their ears. Again, the loss is reversed by removing the foreign object.

Disease processes affecting the tympanic membrane and middle ear cavity are another cause of conductive hearing loss. A perforation of the eardrum, depending upon its size and location, can be responsible for minimal to moderate conductive losses. The loss in this situation may depend upon whether there is a phase difference between the oval and round windows. A perforation over the area of the round window will result in loss of protection to the phase difference and increase the severity of the loss (Fig. 2-10).

In chronic ear disease there may be a combination of pathological processes accounting for the hearing loss. Not only is there a tympanic membrane perforation present but also associated with this may be a va-

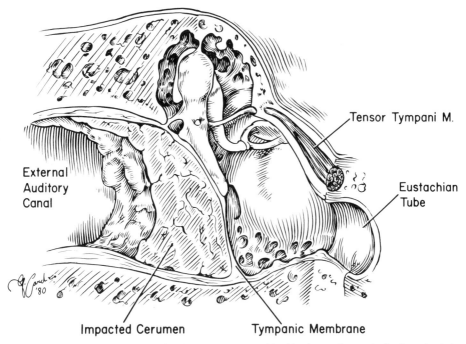

Tensor Tympani M.

External
Auditory
Canal

Eustachian
Tube

Impacted Cerumen   Tympanic Membrane

Figure 2-9. Conductive hearing losses are caused by blockage of sound vibrations in their transfer through the external auditory canal and middle ear. The simplest and one of the commonest forms of conductive hearing loss results from an accumulation of excessive cerumen in the external auditory canal.

riety of ossicular defects. The commonest is necrotic loss of the long process of the incus (Fig. 2-11). A number of possible causes include loss of the superstructure of the stapes and of the handle of the malleus. Destruction of the ossicles may occur as a result of granulation tissue, repeated infections in the tympanic cavity, or cholesteatoma. Skin within the middle ear cleft or mastoid process causes a tremendous amount of destruction over a period of several years. Modern techniques of tympanoplasty, tympanoplasty with mastoidectomy, and methods of ossicular reconstruction make it possible in a high percentage of cases to repair the diseased middle ear and restore hearing.

In some instances the tympanic membrane itself appears normal, but a conductive hearing loss is evident. This situation usually indicates either fixation or discontinuity of the ossicular chain. Impedance audiometry is helpful in distinguishing between the two processes. Discontinuity may be the result of trauma or loss of the long process of the incus. Fixation may occur at the stapes owing to otosclerosis (Fig. 2-12) or a congenital absence of the anular ring of the footplate. Either problem can be corrected

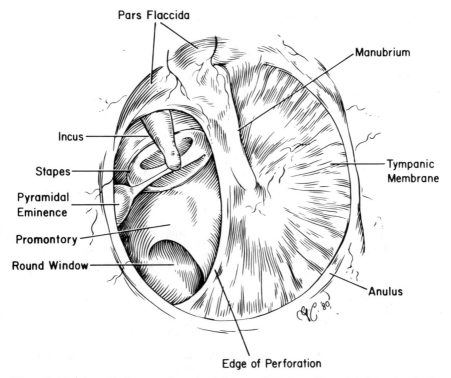

Pars Flaccida

Manubrium

Incus

Stapes

Pyramidal
Eminence

Promontory

Round Window

Tympanic
Membrane

Anulus

Edge of Perforation

Figure 2-10. A perforation over the area of the round window will result in loss of protection to the phase difference and increase the severity of the loss.

by stapedectomy. Occasionally the fixation involves the malleus head and body of the incus, whereas the stapes is freely mobile. This process is usually the result of tympanosclerotic plaques fixing the ossicles in the epitympanum. Hearing can be restored by removing the incus and the head of the malleus followed by reconstruction of the ossicular chain by sculpturing a prosthesis from the incus to fit between the handle of the malleus and the capitulum of the stapes.

Conductive hearing loss commonly occurs behind an intact tympanic membrane. In this situation serous otitis media resulting from eustachian tube malfunction produces a transudate of serous fluid from the mucous membrane lining the middle ear cleft (Fig. 2-13). As the tympanic cavity fills with fluid, the vibrating responses of the tympanic membranes are dampened, thereby creating a conductive loss. In some instances the fluid becomes viscid accounting for the appellation "glue ear." Clear serous fluid can sometimes be removed from the middle ear simply by the Valsalva maneuver. The glue ear will not clear itself in this manner and requires myringotomy and forceful extraction of the material with a suction device.

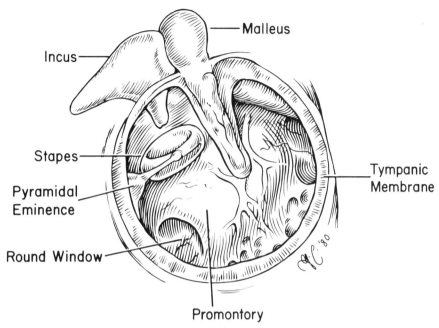

Figure 2-11. In chronic ear disease there may be a combination of pathologic processes accounting for the hearing loss. Not only is there a tympanic membrane perforation present, but associated with this may be a variety of ossicular defects. The commonest is necrotic loss of the long process of the incus.

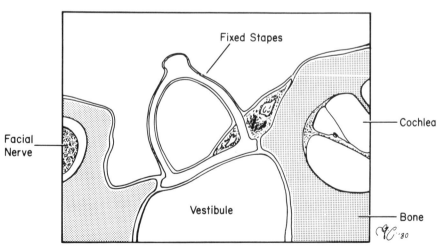

Figure 2-12. In some instances the tympanic membrane itself appears normal but a conductive hearing loss is evident. This situation usually indicates either fixation or discontinuity of the ossicular chain. Impedance audiometry is helpful in distinguishing between the two processes. Discontinuity may be the result of trauma or loss of the long process of the incus. Fixation may occur at the stapes owing to otosclerosis or a congenital absence of the anular ring of the footplate.

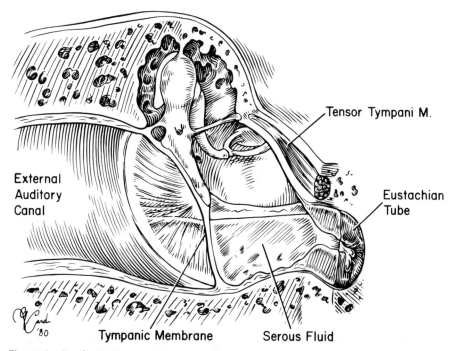

External
Auditory
Canal

Tensor Tympani M.

Eustachian
Tube

Tympanic Membrane   Serous Fluid

Figure 2-13. Conductive hearing loss commonly occurs behind an intact tympanic membrane. In this situation serous otitis media resulting from eustachian tube malfunction produces a transudate of serous fluid from the mucous membrane lining the middle ear cleft.

Recently it has been popular to insert different types of ventilating tubes into the substance of the tympanic membrane to prevent the recurrence of the fluid. The middle ear cleft is ventilated through the plastic tube rather than the patient's eustachian tube. Once the fluid has been removed, and assuming the process does not repeat itself, hearing returns to normal levels.

In summary, conductive hearing losses are, by and large, amenable to some type of surgical intervention.

Sensorineural Hearing Loss

As its name implies, sensorineural or sensory end organ loss occurs when there is damage to or interference with the neural pathways of the auditory system. The conductive mechanism—external auditory canal, tympanic membrane, or ossicular chain—in these cases is usually normal. The cochlear partition is displaced by the movement of the stapes in a routine manner, but electrical impulses created in this manner do not reach the auditory cortex. The lesion may be limited to the hair cell system

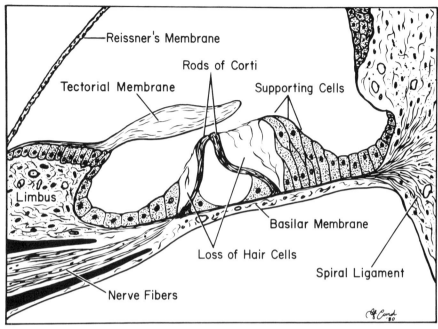

Figure 2-14. Since ototoxic antibiotics are known to destroy hair cells, a patient with a sensorineural loss who is on an antibiotic regimen probably has a sensory loss.

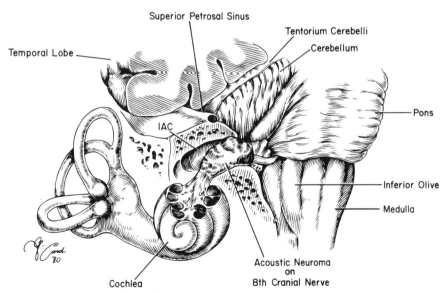

Figure 2-15. The individual with an acoustic tumor most likely would have a neural loss.

(sensory) or to the auditory nerve and central pathways (neural). For practical purposes, losses fitting into this category are not usually defined as to whether they are sensory or neural in nature but are referred to as having a sensorineural loss. If the etiology of the loss is known, it is possible to state with some assurance which type it is. For example, since ototoxic antibiotics are known to destroy hair cells, a patient with a sensorineural loss who is on an antibiotic regimen probably has a sensory loss (Fig. 2–14). The individual with an acoustic tumor, however, would most likely have a neural loss (Fig. 2–15).

The widespread use of E Coch G and BERA make it possible for clinicians to distinguish among the components of a sensorineural loss on a routine basis.

Sensorineural hearing loss may be caused by viral and bacterial infection, head injury or iatrogenic trauma, central nervous system disease such

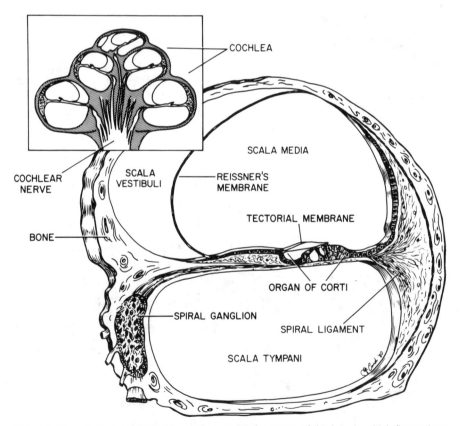

Figure 2–16. Hydrops of the scala media may be the cause of the loss in which fluctuations can often be stabilized by salt restriction and the use of diuretics.

as acoustic tumors and intrinsic brain stem lesions, and as a result of congenital and hereditary defects. One of the most fascinating sensorineural hearing losses is that associated with Meniere's disease. The loss actually fluctuates from one day to another, sometimes by the hour, and will return to normal pure tone levels after an attack. Hydrops of the scala media (Fig. 2-16) may be the cause of the loss, in which case fluctuations can often be stabilized by salt restriction and the use of diuretics. Endolymphatic sac drainage surgery is offered to the individual who does not respond to medical management. If untreated, the process eventually destroys the contents of the cochlear partition, and in many cases the hearing loss progresses to become totally nonresponsive.

At the present state of the art, little if anything can be done to reverse the majority of sensorineural hearing losses, in contrast to conductive losses.

NEUROLOGICAL DISORDERS INVOLVING THE BRAIN STEM

Theoretically, any disease process that is capable of interfering in neural transmission with the central pathways of the auditory system might well produce a sensorineural hearing loss, or at least affect the results of BERA.

Based upon our current knowledge of BERA we may assume that purely cortical (stroke), cerebellar, and extrapyramidal (Parkinson's disease) processes will probably not alter the tracing. Although metabolic (from barbituate administration) and other (hypothermia) problems are alleged not to change BERA, they can alter the test results if the condition is severe enough.

Basically the neurological disorders most commonly associated with abnormal BERA tracings can be divided into two groups: congenital and acquired.

There are primarily three congenital disorders. Prematurity is a common cause. When there is abnormal brain stem development (Moebius syndrome) or abnormal neuroectoderm development (anencephaly hereditary leukodystrophy), the BERA will be altered.

Acquired neurological disorders can be divided into five categories.

Neoplasms

Intensive or extreme neoplasms of the brain stem will almost always alter the BERA. These would include acoustic neuromas, meningiomas, and primary cholesteatomas of the cerebellopontine angle.

Trauma

An individual experiencing a head injury might well develop an epidural, subdural, or intracerebral hemorrhage with lower brain stem compression secondary to central nervous system shift. Fractures of the temporal bone with involvement of the cochlear nerve or middle ear ossicles might cause BERA alterations as well.

Degenerative and Demyelinating Processes

An example of a degenerative process would be the adult form of leukodystrophy. The three most common demyelinating processes that will affect BERA are multiple sclerosis, Schilders diffuse cerebral sclerosis, and hemorrhagic leukoencephalopathies.

Infections

Infections are usually viral and would include anything that would involve white matter in the brain stem such as bulbar poliomyelitis or encephalitis.

Vascular Disorders

A stroke with brain stem involvement caused by difficulty in the basilar artery distribution (either hemorrhagic or ischemic) will cause marked alterations in the BERA.

It is not within the scope of this book to attempt a detailed list of neurological disorders affecting BERA. One must be aware of the fact, however, that a prolonged or absent wave V is not pathopneumonic of an acoustic tumor. The diagnosis of this lesion must be accomplished by means of posterior fossa myelogram or computerized axial tomography (CAT) scanning.

REFERENCES

1. Gray, H.: *Anatomy of the Human Body*. Philadelphia, Lea & Feibeger.
2. Schuknecht, H. F.: *Pathology of the Ear*. Cambridge, Harvard University Press, 1974.
3. Davis, H. F.: Principles of electric response audiometry, *Ann Otol Rhinol Laryngol* 85 (Suppl 28): 1–96, 1976.

4. Schuknecht, H. F.: *Pathology of the Ear*, Cambridge, MA, Harvard University Press, 1974.
5. Rasmussen, G.: Anatomic relationships of the ascending and descending auditory systems. in Fields, W. and Alford, B. (eds.): *Neurological Aspects of Auditory and Vestibular Disorders*. Springfield, IL, Charles C. Thomas, 1964, Chap. I.

Chapter Three

INSTRUMENTATION AND BASIC TECHNIQUE

INTRODUCTION

This chapter is organized to present an overview of the principles and the techniques for brain stem evoked response audiometry as a background for practical applications and is not intended to be a comprehensive explanation of computer analysis procedures. There follows a review of instrumentation, techniques, calibration procedures, and troubleshooting suggestions. Even clinicians concerned primarily with test interpretation rather than test technique should be aware of the following principles.

BIOLOGICAL AVERAGING

Biological averaging allows extraction of a small target signal from random noise. A measurable auditory evoked potential requires synchronous discharge from the cochlea. Such a response can be elicited by a carefully selected stimulus such as a click. Latency of the response to the click depends on sound intensity and the sensitivity of the system being tested.

Principles of Averaging

Signal averaging involves analysis of a number of response samples, amplifying the target response while eliminating other activity or "noise." The background noise at the scalp is the ongoing electroencephalic activity, a relatively large amount of noise in comparison to the small voltage of the brain stem evoked response. The electroencephalic activity produces a random signal with no particular pattern or cycle; that is, it is not time-locked to the onset of the stimulus. When an appropriate acoustic signal is intense enough to evoke an action potential, a small direct current potential is triggered and creates a wave of positive and negative variations relative to the encephelogram (EEG) potentials as the sound-generated impulse completes each neuronal transfer from the cochlea through the auditory nerve and brain stem. Although these events are stable without averaging, these minute electrical changes will be unobservable at the vertex electrode because of the comparatively large voltage of the EEG. The background electrical activity is generally on the order of 10 microvolts, (μv) at the scalp.[1] In contrast, the auditory brain stem responses are on the order of 0.01 to 1 μv.[2] With such a large difference between the noise and the target response signal, observation of a single auditory response is not feasible. The problem, then, is to eliminate "noise" while enhancing the auditory responses. The solution is averaging.

Changes in potential are recorded from the onset of each stimulation to the end of the desired time interval. The averager breaks down this time assignment into "storage bins." In each bin or division the averager stores the relative electrical potential present at that poststimulus time until the run or "epoch" is completed. The averager starts sampling at the instant the click drives the earphone and stops at a set interval after stimulation (for auditory brain stem responses, generally 10 milliseconds [msec] after stimulation). This time period allows evaluation of the brain stem responses in normal adults but must be expanded for some patient responses. Let us assume that the measuring time, called the "gate" or epoch, is 10 msec. At 0 msec the time triggers the stimulus to the cochlea and the computer starts checking each stack or resolution point for storage of the EEG data over the 10-msec period and repeats the procedure until the designated number of sweeps is completed. At the onset of the signal, the sweep begins and stores the data of each time division in a series of rows or columns and repeats this procedure several times. These columns, whose number is determined by computer design, can build above or fall below the relative zero line at each part of a millisecond that the electrical activity is measured. If there is virtually no relative potential at 0.10 msec, that block will be a relatively small contribution to the column. Conversely, continuing with this example, at 5.50 msec a large positive block would be stacked, representing a significant voltage increase, followed at 5.6 msec with a large relative negative voltage. Having stored information for 10 msec the averager will start the collection again at zero, adding voltages in the second run to the columns and so on until the predetermined number of sweeps is reached. Then the averager analyzes the data and provides the arithmetic mean of the data input. If the system being measured is normal, the response will appear as five to seven "bumps," generally designated as the Jewett[3] sequence. This straight-line average with no signal and the resulting change with auditory response are shown in Figures 3-1 and 3-2.

Since the gate is synchronized only to the acoustical signal, random electrical noise such as the ongoing cortical activity, movement, myo-

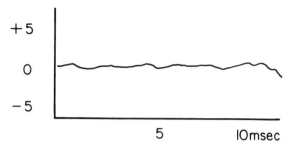

Figure 3-1. Example of average of random activity (no sound). Line represents averaged activity to ±0.5 volts for 1024 samples at eight samples per second, with the subject asleep.

graphic response, and so on will be averaged to zero. Current computer technique is such that time-locked responses add in a linear fashion, whereas random responses add as the square root of the number of stimulations. That is, repeating the sweep 100 times will result in a 10:1 signal-to-noise improvement. Thus, at very large samples, most computer systems can add only a small increase in the signal-to-noise ratio, and for some equipment the desired response actually becomes blunted in the additional averaging.

Averagers store the information digitally. In most clinically designed systems at present the signals are coded by analogue and are converted to digital code in the A-to-D converter, so that the voltages are stored as two-digit numbers. Conversion is made for each point of evaluation during the preset time for every run and is averaged at the conclusion. To obtain

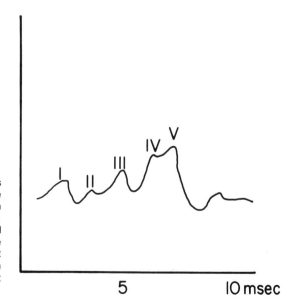

Figure 3-2. Same conditions as in Figure 3-1, except that the average is time-locked to an acoustical stimulus, a click (0.1 msec at 50 dB above threshold for the stimulus). These baseline changes in the average represent the early auditory brain stem responses known as the Jewett sequence.

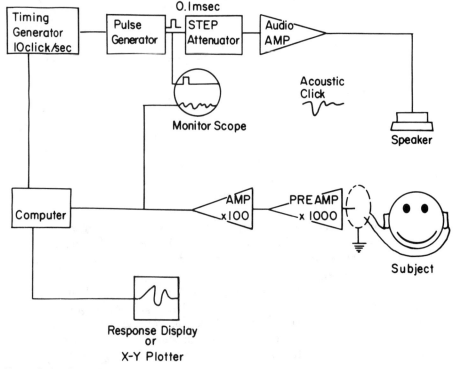

Figure 3–3. Block diagram for recording auditory evoked potentials.

sufficient analysis, 12-bit amplitude resolution is considered sufficient, and the averager should provide time base 256 words of a 24-bit length.

In summary, the purpose of averaging is simply to enhance the target response while minimizing background noise. Ability to detect the brain stem auditory responses is also dependent on proper instrumentation and test technique. Figure 3–3 outlines some of the sections that will be discussed below.

INSTRUMENTATION

Preamplifier

The preamplifier applies the principle of common mode rejection (CMR) for further enhancement of the signal. In a differential amplifier, voltages observed at the active electrode are subtracted from those at the reference or indifferent electrode by reversing its polarity. The result is cancellation of all voltage activity common to both electrodes and through this CMR the target signal becomes the primary electrical input for amplification and data storage. CMR allows cancellation of such artifacts as 60-cycle interference or random internal responses. The ability of the equipment to provide such a function is expressed as the "CMR ratio," the ratio of the two outputs when some specified signal is applied. A high rejection rate is desirable.

Because the preamplifier has the task of boosting the signal on the order of 10^6, its own internal noise characteristics must be known. The internal noise level is determined by measuring noise present when the preamplifier leads are shorted. Since it is impossible to eliminate preamplifier noise completely, the best compromise is a preamplifier that is specified to have low internal noise. As high input impedance is also desirable, there is a certain amount of trade-off involved. Generally 10 μv peak-to-peak internal noise with 50 megohms input impedance is acceptable.

In addition to providing CMR and a relatively quiet boost of the target signal, the preamplifier improves the auditory response through filtering. Most amplifiers are designed with broad frequency response, normally 1 Hertz (Hz) to 10 kilohertz (kHz). If the system's frequency response is altered to filter out undesired noise in low- and high-frequency ranges containing little or no auditory responses, the resulting average will be easier to analyze. Clinical studies[4-6] suggest 3 kHz (3 decibels [dB]down) as the high cutoff, but there is less agreement regarding a low pass setting. Coats and Martin[4] suggest 50 Hz, Jerger and colleagues[5] 300 Hz, and Selters and Brackmann[6] 30 Hz. This variation depends in part on other response characteristics of the equipment in use and in part on the information desired in the average. In our experience the auditory brain stem responses are enhanced with 50 or 100 Hz low pass.

Finally, since the preamplifier must also provide patient protection to minimize shock hazard, clinical units are designed to isolate the patient from the instrument power.

Digital Section

The filtered amplified analogue signal is fed from the preamplifier to the digital section of the averager, where it is stored in the memory. In the A-to-D converter it is possible to provide artifact rejection, so that maximum use of the memory will be available to retain relevant signals instead of averaging noise. Artifact rejection simply involves discarding any sweeps with a specified number of off-scale points. Some clinical units use a preset, often at 5 percent. Others vary the acceptable percentage of off-scale points. In difficult situations it may be possible to obtain a recognizable Jewett series, even though some off-scale data are allowed into the averager. One of our subjects, a patient with chronic spasms of the neck muscles, provided noisy but identifiable, repeatable responses with only artifact rejection eliminated from the system. With artifact rejection at 5 percent, too few acceptable responses were obtained after 5 minutes of attempts at 10 pulses per second (pps) to complete a sample of 512 responses. However, if no response can be observed under these conditions, it is not possible to make any interpretation of the results. Artifact rejection is an important asset in eliminating test artifact noise, though flexibility is desirable.

The digital section stores the voltages as a series of binary numbers called "bits," which represent each sample point and stores them as "words." To provide sufficient amplitude resolution for signal conversion, 12 bits are desirable. The averager takes these digitized data into the memory, where a true arithmetic average is maintained. Sufficient memory is provided by a unit with 24 bits with a minimum of 256 A-to-D conversion points. Some clinical units also provide for splitting the memory so that more than one run can be retained and superimposed for verification of retest of the response. In the averager there is a final conversion of the stored digital information to analogue form for display on an oscilloscope.

Recorders

There are several methods for permanent recording of the response. They can be retained in digital form on computer tape. In most clinical settings, however, it is more practical to record the oscilloscope signal with a strip chart recorder or X-Y plotter. Some clinicians have employed a camera—a slow process but useful in special situations such as the operating room.

Stimulus Section

Another major phase of instrumentation is the stimulus section. For acquisition of clinically useful responses, the stimulus must be capable of provoking synchronous discharge of a large number of fibers. A signal producing such a large action potential must have a rapid rise time. Several types of signals are capable of producing enough response synchrony to yield a visible Jewett sequence. The pure tone stimulus produced by standard clinical audiometers has such a slow rise time that cochlear response is too desynchronized to be visible in the ongoing activity. A click, however, readily produced with a fast rise time (1 msec or less)[1], can elicit a response easily averaged out of the ongoing EEG. Synchrony is achieved both by onset characteristics and by frequency components. The stimulus must contain sufficient high-frequency energy to initiate discharge from the basal turn of the cochlea. Responses from the lower-frequency ranges of the medical and apical regions of the cochlea are less reliable or to desynchronous to be extracted directly from the other neuroelectrical potential. An example of such a stimulus is shown in Figure 3-4.

Currently there are several types of stimuli that will provide good BERA data:

1. *The broad band click or square wave.* This stimulus meets the need for fast rise time and since it has a broad frequency range of energy, it will stimulate the high-frequency region important for a recordable brain stem response. Its duration must be as brief as possible, well under 1 msec, for use in averaged response audiometry. Although its electrical wave form is that of a rectangular pulse, the acoustic response will have peaks reflecting the transducer characteristics.

2. *Filtered clicks.* These stimuli are also easily produced and are more specific in stimulation. They are generated by ringing a third-octave bandpass filter with a raw click or single sine wave. Click duration is a function of the filter frequency. The advantage of filtering is the production of more selective frequency stimulation, which is important in threshold BERA.

3. *Tone pips.* These signals are another alternative with adequate rise time characteristics and frequency specificity. The signal is a pure tone gated to control rise time and plateau for a given frequency, so that it produces a narrow peak at the indicated frequency as measured at the transducer. Davis[1] described use of this stimulus down to 1000 Hz to predict audiometric response curve.

4. *Single cycle pip.* This variant is formed by gating the tone from peak to peak to produce rapid rise time with tone-specific character. This signal is technically more difficult to produce but is less affected by transducer characteristics.

5. *Logon.* The Gaussian logon is a pure tone that is amplitude-modulated across a Gaussian distribution curve and is the best compromise between ideal frequency and rapid rise time according to Davis.[1] The logon is produced as a brief pip gated on and off over the distribution curve, so that it is much like a filtered click and acoustically it presents a broad peak at the pip frequency.

The stimulus generator should also provide control of signal polarity. In difficult recording sites, the polarity of the signal can be alternated to obtain cancellation of artifact and cochlear microphonic (CM). Because there are special situations in which observation of the microphonic is

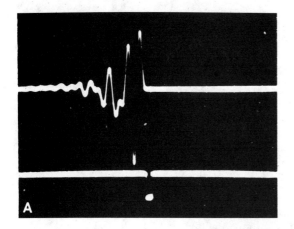

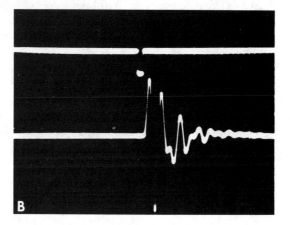

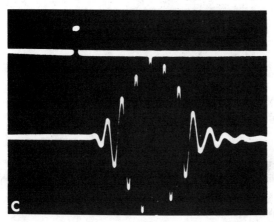

Figure 3-4. *A* and *B,* Representations of electrical and acoustical output to a click (Life-tech 8101 AR mainframe/click generator model 8042 Life-tech model 8049 shielded headphones coupled to artificial ear, click width = 0.1 ms. *C,* A 4 kHz 1 ms msec/fall with 0.1 msec hold time.

desirable, the stimulus section should provide the capability of alternating polarity and providing a choice of compression or rarefaction phases. It should be noted that response interpretation will be significantly affected by this variable, and latency data will vary depending on choice of polarity.

Since stimulus characteristics are variable and are not standardized for BERA, reports of such criteria as normal range of latency and other response data must be understood as peculiar to that laboratory and not directly transferable to another set of circumstances. That is, latency and amplitude data cannot be compared from one clinic to another without concession to differences in instrumentation and procedure. Table 3-1 gives some idea of the range variability of stimuli employed by different investigators.

The stimulus section must also provide a means of intensity control. The intensity is variably specified in terms of reference to a normal jury of hearers or in terms of peak equivalent sound pressure level (peSPL) with 0.0002 microbar reference. The upper limit of available power is determined in part by the nature of the stimulus and the transducer, but should be on the order of 130 dB peSPL and should allow variation downward to O dB peSPL to allow for threshold testing and other intensity variation procedures. (Techniques for determining output are suggested under the section on calibration.)

The stimulus section should include a time to activate the averager simultaneously with the stimulus onset. It should allow variation in repetition rate from sufficiently slow, to allow adequate recovery—generally under 20 pulses per second, to rapid for both site of lesion and threshold

TABLE 3-1. Stimulus Variations in Several BERA Laboratories

Source	Stimulus
Selters and Brackmann[6]	160 microsec DC pulse applied 20 pps to earphones
Mokotoff, Schulmann-Galambos, Galambos[7]	0.1 msec square wave
Stockard and Rossiter[8]	Acoustic transients 0.1 msec
Starr and Hamilton[9]	"Clicks"
Davis[1]	Brief (0.2 msec or less) click at 1.2 and 4 Hz tone pips
Coats and Martin[4]	0.02 msec square wave pulse
Clemis and McGee[10]	Tone pip 1 msec rise and decoy with total duration 2 msec (no plateau)
Glasscock et al.[11]	0.1 msec click (see Fig. 3-4).

procedures. Note that since the stimuli are below critical duration, threshold is achieved at greater intensity than for a stimulus of standard duration matched in frequency. Direct inferences of threshold based on peSPL must take this difference into account. The basis for selecting repetition rate is presented later in this chapter.

Finally, the stimulus section includes the transducer. The stimulus can drive a free-field speaker, although this complicates monitoring intensity of signal at the eardrum, or it can be presented through an earphone. Since the response characteristics of the standard TDH 49 earphone can affect the high-frequency character of the stimulus, other earspeakers are sometimes preferred. For special test problems, a bone conduction transducer is a helpful addition. (See Chapter 3.)

Electrodes

A final consideration in instrumentation is the link of the patient to the preamplifier. The response generated by the appropriately prescribed stimulus must be detected for delivery to the preamplifier. The sensors, scalp electrodes, pick up the preliminary scalp potentials including EEG noise, artifact and auditory potential. Most commonly, gold or silver-silver chloride discs acting as volume conductors applied with reduced skin resistance (generally under 5000 ohms) will provide adequate signal input. The electrodes sense response of the various auditory generators, acting as dipoles, depending on their proximity and relative signal strength. If the dipole is oriented toward the electrode, the measured discharge will appear greater. That is, if the active electrode is at the vertex in parallel with the electrical potential changes, the response will have the greatest volume. As opposed to some electroencephalographic procedures, the monopolar technique for recording auditory response results in less distortion than bipolar measures.[12]

In summary, instrumentation requires an appropriate stimuli to elicit a detectable response at the surface electrodes. This signal is boosted and refined in the preamplifier, is converted to numerical date for averaging, and is stored in the digital section with final reproduction to visual representation on the oscilloscope.

TECHNIQUE

Introduction

Brain stem audiometric technique varies, depending on the purpose of the procedure—either site of lesion assessment or threshold determination.

This section will describe some of the techniques of response acquisition and analysis.

Electrodes

There are several successful techniques for application and placement of electrodes to eliminate the problems of noise and poor retest. It is important to place the active electrode in the vicinity of C_z, the vertex. It can be located by intersecting lines joining nasion to inion and the preauricular points. The amplitude of the responses and polarity will vary depending on the relative position of the active electrode. For best analysis of the Jewett sequence, the electrode should approximate C_z although a slight variation has a limited effect. There are advocates of forehead placement for the active site to avoid problems of placing the electrode in hair, but this procedure distorts responses of the fourth- and fifth-order neurons (wave V). Since wave V in a normal subject has large amplitude, it vill be visible with active electrode at the forehead. However, in a patient with an abnormally decreased response amplitude, the response may appear to be absent or less repeatable with such an angled placement. Figure 3-5 compares forehead and vertex responses from a patient diagnosed as having multiple sclerosis and demonstrates distortion.

Although the active electrode needs to be seated at the vertex for maximum amplitude of wave V, successful placement of the reference electrode varies. Sites include the ipsilateral mastoid, earlobe (front or back), and neck. None is truly indifferent, though the earlobe tends to have the least active participation. In our experience, neck placement has proved a problem because of neuromuscular potentials. In general, the ipsilateral site is the reference, and the contralateral pair serves as the ground. Some investigators add a fourth electrode as a ground, placed equidistant between right and left references and roughly perpendicular to the line of travel of the auditory potential. The nasion is a common choice for the site; however, in our experience the addition of the fourth electrode has not improved clinical interpretation or response reliability over pairing with the opposite site.

Sufficient reduction in skin resistance can be achieved by cleansing and abrading the scalp and taping electrodes filled with a conducting gel to the prepared surface. The more traditional technique from EEG laboratories involves abrading through a perforated electrode after it is sealed to the skin or scalp with collodion. Collodion-fixed electrodes will remain stable for hours. The "pasting" technique requires less abrasion to the scalp and less equipment and will provide adequate resistance reduction for less time, 1 to 2 hours generally. It is important to test the electrodes for adequate reduction of skin resistance to 3000 to 5000 ohms or less. Also, balancing of interelectrode resistance is important in eliminating large differences as well as attempting to gain low impedances to make CMR effective.[13] However, under adverse conditions we have recorded responses from electrodes at 9000 ohms, but we have also balanced resistance.

Pitfalls

There are some other special considerations with electrode placement. The following suggestions are based on our experience with more than 1000 recordings in the course of which a number of pitfalls were encountered.

1. *Reference placement problems.* There are some practical considerations in choosing the reference location. Old mastoid bowls are poor sites, both because of difficulty in attaching the electrode cup to the pitted area and because of comparatively poor conductivity of the underlying tissue. Scarred or keratomatous earlobes are also poor conductors. In both cases an alternative site is recommended.

2. *Protection from the transducer.* If the earspeaker is employed, it may dislodge the electrode, particularly if it is placed on the outside surface of the earlobe. Placing it on the mastoid process or the mesial surface of the earlobe generally provides the protection of the pinna when the earphone is in place. The mesial surface of the earlobe is more neutral and is not in direct contact with the transducer cover; it is also less comfortable and occasionally cannot be tolerated long enough to complete the procedure.

3. *Access for placement.* The front surface of the pinna provides easy access even on a sleeping or anesthetized patient. The tissue has relatively low natural resistance, though the electrodes are occasionally dislodged by contact with the earphone cushions.

4. *Patient artifacts.* If scar tissue is present at the active electrode site, placement should be varied to accommodate or avoid it. Of course the active electrode provides unacceptable contact if attached through a toupee, but there will also be excessive resistance over a hair transplant. A plastic surgical prosthesis increases resistance to potential transfer, and a prosthesis creates a huge artifact. In one patient, evaluation of asymmetrical hearing loss went on for more than an hour without obtaining proper recording conditions before the patient mentioned that he had a right temporal bone prosthesis. We obtained a BERA measurement by using neck tissue on both sides with the anticipated but manageable neuromuscular artifact introduced by this placement. Another potential problem is scalp dandruff or psoriasis, since psoriatic detritus is a distinctly poor electrical conductor. It is advisable to clean the area carefully with a cosmetic sponge to reach the scalp and provide a good electrode field. In general, electrode

placement should accomodate any special patient problems to provide low scalp-skin resistance and roughly equal interelectrode balance.

Patient State

The next step in administering BERA is to provide a good test environment. The primary consideration is the subject's state of relaxation. Generally, adults will cooperate sufficiently to provide an ongoing EEG on the order of 10^5 μv. If the environment is restful and the patient can lie down, the record will generally be quiet enough. Because of the monotony of the click stimuli, many subjects will sleep, providing ideal recording. Although it is certainly helpful to test the patient in quiet, since noise will reduce response amplitude and make patient relaxation more difficult, room noise like that of an intensive care unit or surgical theater does not preclude successful suprathreshold administration of the test.

Response latencies are not affected by depth of sleep, sedation, anesthesia, or by any other drug at nontoxic levels. Starr and Achor[14] reported excellent clinical results even with patients in drug coma and Stockard and Jones[15] found effects of drug or anesthesia only at massive doses. In particular the anticonvulsants at therapeutic levels had no effects. Tranquilizers, including the families of phenothiazenes, benzodiazipines, and short-acting barbiturates, had no effect even at toxic doses (in cats). In several cases of toxic doses in humans, only one patient showed abnormal response, but his hypothermia was considered to be a critical factor affecting latency.[15] Steroids and antimicrobials even at mass doses in cats had no effect. Squires and colleaques[16] found that alcohol (ethanol) intoxication may prolong central conduction time in cats; data for humans are not available. Stockard and Jones[15] also reported that neither isoflurane nor barbiturates abolished brain stem responses when administered concentrations were well above levels maintained for a deep level of anesthesia. Enflurane did not abolish the response, but for unknown reasons later response components were affected selectively during the recovery phase. Other investigators have also reported no drug effect. Davis[1] has reported clinical use of secobarbital without effect; Stockard and Rossiter[8] have described patients with diazepam-induced relaxation, and Jerger and colleagues[5] have reported good results with chloral hydrate. Halothane (fluorane) anesthesia has been used with children in our population and has provided normal central conduction time in 10 of 12 patients who required anesthesia for the procedure. One of the two patients with abnormal conduction time had no response at all and subsequent polytomography revealed abnormal cochlear structure. A second patient had prolonged conduction from wave I to wave V and had several other indications of brain stem abnormality. Based on literature and our own experience, halothane anesthesia provides an excellent recording condition without biasing response characteristics. Ketamine is also popular in some sections of the country for anesthesia with pediatric patients, although there are undocumented reports that the agent can affect response. Because the drug sometimes has undesirable side effects in children, primarily in terms of its hallucinogenic nature, our anesthesiologists do not suggest its use routinely.

It is important to stress that drugs are seldom needed to obtain the desired response, but the patient can be tested under the influence of drugs, conscious or unconscious, with minimal effect on early auditory responses.

Some patients with neuromuscular disorders, arthritis, or anxiety will require special relaxation techniques. For straightforward psychological or physical tension, the physician may choose to administer a muscle relaxant or sedative. In rare cases, allowing the patient to submit to testing seated instead of in the customary supine position will provide adequate relaxation. Certainly, poor test response calls for a thorough analysis of test conditions. A 28-year-old female who presented with multiple otological complaints, including hearing loss and vertigo, appeared apprehensive but cooperative during attempts to obtain auditory evoked responses. At the beginning of each measurement the patient response was quiet, but marked break-up consistent with neuromuscular activity eventually interrupted the run. The patient was requested to relax and maintain a quiet state, but with no improvement in the recording. On close observation we noted that the patient repeatedly dropped her head to the right shoulder and could not prevent this chronic sagging. Diazepam was administered and subsequently obtained evoked potentials were found to be normal, although the patient was in early stages of a neuromuscular disease of unknown etiology. Figure 3–6 indicates the difference between premedication and postmedication evoked potentials on the right ear.

Pediatric and uncooperative patients pose another challenge in creating a good test environment. Most children, even infants, can be tested if the examiner is patient and flexible with them. Some, however, do not provide reliable recordings in a reasonable amount of time without sedation. Although an audiologist may consider the need for sedation or anesthesia, decisions about how much and what kind must be made by a physician. Since patients who are hard to test are either often very young (less than age 3 years) or have multiple physical problems, the potential for adverse response may well increase in this group, compared to the average subject receiving the same dose. For this reason, it is strongly recommended that such special test conditions as sedation or drug-induced sleep be provided when an attending physician and emergency equipment are available. In our experience one subject with a functional component to his

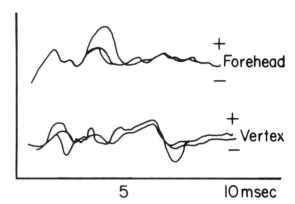

Figure 3-5. Example of varying active electrode placement on a patient with abnormal response, active at forehead in top three traces, at Cz on lower three traces. Reference to ipsilateral mastoid, at 60 dB above patient threshold for click, 8 pps.

hearing loss had to be sedated for BERA because he gritted his teeth for the initial test session. Sedation was ordered by the physician and shortly after administration (intramuscular and oral), it was possible to establish the degree of peripheral deficit in the high frequencies with a good retest. It should be stressed that the decision to provide sedatives was medical and that it was administered when constant supervision against potential adverse reactions was present.

Before drugs are considered, the clinician should attempt to obtain BERA without them, even with a pediatric subject. Infants will sleep if a parent can delay their nap time for the procedure and bring a hungry child to the test suite with bottle, blanket, and teddy bear or anything that will suggest naptime. Older children in the toddler category (roughly 12 to 36 months) may or may not cooperate in a reasonable amount of time. If a child in this age range cannot be assessed by more conventional techniques it is possible that he also cannot relax adequately for reliable BERA. If they are to undergo other procedures such as radiological studies, general anesthesia for the combined procedures may be warranted. This application of BERA is warranted only in cases in which peripheral auditory response cannot be determined by other procedures. This application will be discussed in detail in Chapter 4.

In summary, although most patients will provide good response without special techniques, it is sometimes necessary to sedate or anesthetize the patient. The response is unaffected by patient state.

Repetition Rate

Repetition rate is a significant instrumentation variable. Site of lesion studies are obtained at a relatively slow repetition rate (20 pulses per second or less). Our laboratory uses 8 pulses per second for routine studies.

TABLE 3–2. Repetition Rate Suggested in Various BERA Laboratories

REPETITION RATE	
Selters and Brackmann[6]	20 pps
Stockard and Rossiter[8]	10 pps
Starr and Hamilton[9]	10 per sec
Mokotoff et al.[7]	33.3
Jerger et al.[5]	20
Davis[1]	20
Glasscock et al.[11]	8
Coats and Martin[4]	20
Fria and Sabo[17]	10 to 30 pps
Starr and Achor[14]	8

Table 3-2 samples several reports of BERA for repetition rate. Repetition rate is important because an adequate interstimulus interval is necessary for baseline recording. Eggermont and colleagues[18] found the eighth nerve action potential was markedly affected as the interstimulus interval was shortened below critical refractory period. Figure 3-7 illustrates the problems related to data collection at rapid repetition rates. This normal subject illustrates responses consistent with the report by Weber and Fujikawa[19] who found that repetition rate significantly affects intensity-latency functions in normal subjects. Theoretically, pathological ears should also show changes as rate increases but the patterns are not well documented. For clinical purposes it is important to use a sufficiently slow repetition rate so that the response is easily observed and subject to retest. The increase in test time at a slow rate is warranted in view of the more repeatable latency and improved detail of the response. However, faster repetition rates are useful in expediting threshold testing since a restless infant can be screened by rapid stimulation during the quiet periods that are available. The examiner can screen for wave V at fast rates, up to 40 pulses per second,

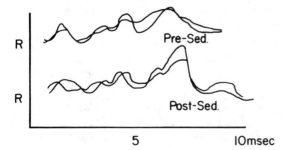

Figure 3-6. Two representative runs on a patient in chronic muscle spasm. Upper curves (without sedation) are difficult to analyze and present poor retest. Lower wave forms show responses (normal) from this same patient after oral administration of diazepam.

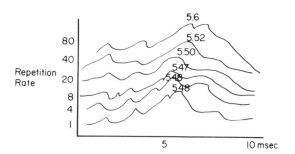

Figure 3-7. Illustration of increasing repetition rate for BERA with normal subject. Note both latency shift and loss of detail at high rates. N = 1024, I = 85 peSPL with 0.1 msec click.

although once the threshold can be estimated, slow runs are necessary to extract the lower-amplitude wave V.

There are also reports using very rapid stimulus repetition to look at adaptation of evoked potentials. As demonstrated in Figure 3-7, responses in a normal subject show change in latency. As suggested by Thornton and Coleman's data,[20] a normal subject will demonstrate a latency increase adaptation apparently by cumulative loss at low and relatively high brain stem levels. There is the suggestion by Daly and colleagues[21] that an increase in repetition rate will aid in defining auditory pathology. The application of such techniques to documented pathology at varying levels of the auditory system is necessary before such data can be incorporated into routine clinical procedure. At present, there is insufficient information to distinquish the level of pathology with rapid repetition rates. These rates may be useful in threshold tests.

Size of Sample

The number of samples per patient depends in part on computer design and more importantly on the purpose of the procedure. Increasing the

TABLE 3–3. Number of Samples Per Run Suggested in Several BERA Laboratories

Reference	Samples per Average
Selters and Brackmann[6]	1000
Mokotoff et al.[7]	1024 to 4096
Stockard and Rossiter[8]	2000 to 4000
Starr and Hamilton[9]	2048
Coats and Martin[4]	1000
Glasscock et al.[11]	1000

number of runs reduces the noise level, but improvement in response visibility is less as large collection levels are reached. Most clinical reports suggest that 1024 to 2048 averages are sufficient for site-of-lesion procedures, whereas others use as many as 4000. Some of the variations are summarized in Table 3-3. In threshold testing the average needs to continue only long enough to determine the latency of wave V. At high intensity under good conditions this response may be evident after only 256 sweeps. Threshold procedures should vary the number of samples to obtain adequate response as efficiently as possible. As the intensity approaches the threshold, more samples are required to determine wave V latency than at suprathreshold levels. For this reason sample at suspected threshold should include a relatively large average, at least 1024. For most clinical applications 2048 runs reach the upper limit of practical reduction of noise through repetition, and 1024 is often sufficient.

Stimulus Intensity

Stimulus intensity is another important variable. Peak latency of wave V is not achieved until 40 to 60 dB above threshold. Response amplitude may increase with intensity growth, but latency will not diminish above this point. As intensity is decreased, wave V latency will increase until threshold is reached (Fig. 3-8). Wave V is the most persistent auditory brain stem response and is still recordable near voluntary threshold, whereas recording of the entire Jewett sequence requires supra-

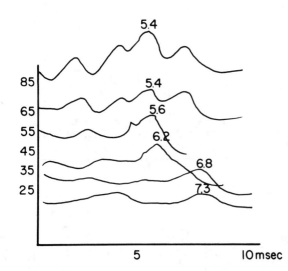

Figure 3-8. Latency-intensity function in a normal-hearing subject. As intensity is increased, amplitude increases and latency decreases.

threshold testing. There is also a marked improvement in amplitude with increased intensity. Some site-of-lesion reports[6,8,14] suggest sampling at one intensity only. Others [11,22] vary intensity according to degree of loss. Central conduction time is easier to analyze at a relatively loud presentation level (roughly 40 to 60 dB over stimulus threshold), but identification is severely complicated near threshold. Interpretation of site-of-lesion tests based on latency of wave V without regard to sensation level of the signal runs the risk of unnecessary false-positive response readings. The stimulus must provoke high-frequency response to provide sufficient synchrony for a visible wave V. Practically speaking, the sound must be above action potential threshold by a minimum of 40 dB in a normal system to reach the most efficient wave V. For a patient with high-frequency loss, interpretation of the averaged response at arbitrary stimulation level is unnecessarily difficult. The sound intensity should be manipulated to accommodate hearing loss, so that sufficient data are available to evaluate central conduction time or at least to determine whether an increase in intensity will decrease the latency of wave V. The alternative is to hold intensity constant[6] and to interpret the latency of wave V with regard to the degree of loss with a formula based on clinical findings of proven cochlear lesions of known loss.

Generally site-of-lesion evaluation should begin at a relatively loud level (40 to 60 dB above average threshold for the stimulus in normal subjects). For site-of-lesion test patients, the audiogram will allow a prediction of required stimulus intensity or will suggest possible compromise of test interpretation because of the severity of the loss. Since the test stimulus is not a standard audiometric signal, it is useful to establish voluntary threshold for the test stimulus. When patient thresholds for the stimuli are not obtainable, the formula and statistical data of Selters and Brackmann[6] and Jerger and colleagues[5] provide an indirect interpolation of acceptable latency of wave V. If wave I can also be determined, central conduction time will make retrocochlear site-of-lesion test interpretation independent of stimulus intensity. Variation of intensity in 10 dB steps from threshold to earliest wave V latency will also yield a latency-intensity function that is helpful in separating conductive from cochlear lesions as will be described in Chapter 4. Steep latency functions are consistent with cochlear disorder[5], whereas functions that are displaced but parallel to normal represents conductive hearing loss.

A latency-intensity curve is also established in threshold testing. Since wave amplitude is a function of stimulus intensity, it is advisable to begin the procedure well above the estimated threshold, where wave V is relatively easy to identify. The threshold of wave V in ideal test conditions is also highly repeatable, though it is much smaller in amplitude, and latency is increased (Fig. 3-8).

Preamplifier Filters

Filter settings also affect the auditory responses, most prominently in amplitude. Many clinicians agree on 3000 Hz as the high-frequency setting, since there is relatively little significant information above that frequency range, but noise in the recording is somewhat increased (Fig. 3–9). There is much less agreement on low-frequency setting, since there is a significant increase in noise as the setting is lowered (Fig. 3–10). Since the auditory responses vary in latency and morphology as the low-frequency cut-off is changed, it is important to maintain a constant low-frequency setting for comparison of the patient response to normal subjects in interpreting evoked potential. For example, changing the filter from 50 to 300 Hz to eliminate noise will preclude interpreting wave V latency in terms of the normative data established at 50 Hz. It is helpful to filter out low-frequency noise in difficult situations such as testing in an intensive care unit, but the examiner must be aware that the response is biased. Ordinarily, an effectively quiet recording can be obtained with a low-frequency

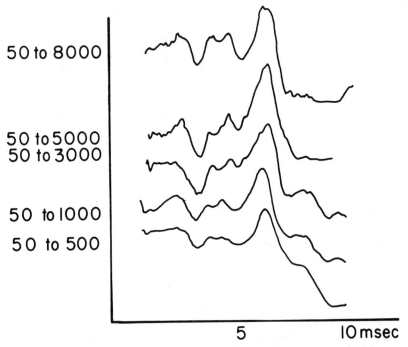

Figure 3–9. Effect of altering high-frequency filter for auditory evoked potentials on a normal-hearing subject. Low-pass setting is held constant at 50 Hz. Detail is distorted at 1 kHz and lower, but little is added as filter is set above 3 kHz. (1024 samples at 85 peSPL, 0.1 msec click).

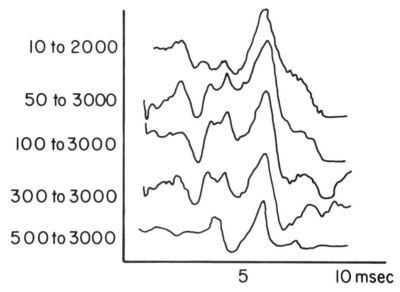

10 to 2000

50 to 3000

100 to 3000

300 to 3000

500 to 3000

5   10 msec

Figure 3-10. Effect of altering low-frequency filter for auditory evoked potentials on a normal-hearing subject. High-pass setting is held constant at 3000 Hz. Noise increases significantly at 50 Hz and lower. However, response detail is somewhat better at 100 Hz and lower (1024 samples, 85 peSPL, 0.1 msec).

filter setting of 50 or 100 Hz. In summary, filters should be varied to accommodate the test environment, but response interpretation should be documented by a knowledge of normal responses with those filter settings.

Stimulus Characteristics

The stimulus must have a rapid rise time and frequency energy to provoke a synchronous discharge. Some clinical stimulus generators allow the examiner to vary signal characteristics. For site-of-lesion procedures, the high-frequency brief duration settings provide maximal amplitude with more precise wave peaks, making the recording easier to analyze. At frequencies below 1000 cycles the tone is stimulating a relatively broad segment of the basilar membrane toward the apical turn of the cochlea, with the result that the desynchronous response is difficult or impossible to analyze reliably.[1] This procedure does not allow for sampling response through the entire frequency range for hearing, but it is possible to obtain averages with the stimulus frequency range approximating 1000 Hz. Wave V thresholds are not as repeatable at low frequency as they are in higher ranges nor do they approximate voluntary thresholds as closely as at higher frequencies, at which the wave V threshold is highly retestable at an average of 10 dB over voluntary threshold for normal subjects. Alternative methods for inferring the low-frequency threshold have been tried and are reviewed in Chapter 4.

Because different types of stimuli are in use, it is important to define the stimulus as precisely as possible. Specifying the electrical impulse only is not completely adequate, since the transducer modification is generally considerable. The stimulus is defined much better if the acoustical spectrum of the signal is also presented.

Stimulus Phase

Another signal characteristic that affects the response is stimulus phase. Alternating polarity will eliminate the early electrical and mechanical artifacts in averaging along with the CM, though it will not affect the compound action potential. However, averaging both condensation and rarefaction waves will have the effect of desynchronizing the response, since these two phases will have slightly different timing in stimulating the cochlea. There is a small error or variation in wave latency in comparing rarefaction with condensation stimuli, since this phase shift will cause a slightly different generation of the action potential and may or may not be apparent upon averaging, depending on the nature of the timelock of stimulus and averager. Coats and Martin[4] found that in high-frequency loss rarefaction responses were out of phase with condensation runs at waves II through IV, whereas there was little difference at wave V. They suggest that there are two components in the response, that is, two parallel pathways, with waves III, IV, and VI representing one pathway and V a different route. Pending further clinical investigation as to the origin of this difference, the important factor here is to settle upon a consistent choice of polarity to eliminate this additional source of variation.

Masking

The use of masking to prevent crossover of the stimulus to the nontest ear is standard protocol for most test procedures. Masking is also important in determining whether the right or left pathways are under test in evoked response audiometry. Masking desynchronizes response of the opposite ear to minimize its contribution. Interaural attenuation is relatively large, roughly 60 dB for a stimulus exciting regions higher than 3000 Hz, which is the range of most site of lesion stimuli. Whether contralateral masking is present or not, off-side responses should be suspected when markedly abnormal patterns are present. If a crossover response appears, its latencies should be those of stimuli approximately 60 dB lower than the intensity to the opposite ear. Remarkably, this crossover is not always seen. Further studies are certainly needed to define masking more precisely.

If the response is off-side, amplitude will be comparatively poor. Suppose, for instance, the clinician knows nothing about the patient, he presents the clicks to the right ear and obtains a threshold of 20 dB peSPL at 0.1 msec. If the opposite ear yields no response until 90 dB at 8.2 msec, is the wave crossover or representative of left ear response? Desynchronizing the opposite ear with masking in this case will eliminate participation of the off-side ear. It may also damp the amplitude of the target response somewhat. When possibile crossover problems complicate data interpretation, the clinician may want to consider impedance audiometry, E Coch G, or BERA with bone-conducted stimuli (See Chap. 5).

Patient Variables

Amplitude and latency are somewhat sex-dependent. Stockard and colleagues[23] recommend maintaining latency data by sex for close examination of responses. In reviewing BERA for 20 young female and 20 young male subjects (less than age 30 years) in our group, the mean latency of wave V was 0.15 msec later in men, although there was overlap in the ranges. Although this small group and the unspecified population in the study by Stockard and coworkers[23] suggests a sex-related difference in latency, further analysis of the test variable is needed to confirm this tendency. Sex may also influence amplitude, since this measure has been described as larger in the young female.[23] Certainly it is easy to demonstrate a dramatic Jewett wave V on a young cooperative female. In a review of 20 male and 20 female patients with normal responses in our clinic, amplitude was compared by measuring voltage from maximum positive to maximum negative in waves I, III, and V. Although wave I and III amplitudes were virtually interchangeable in comparing the two groups, wave V averaged 12.7 per cent larger for females than for those in the male group, with a range of −4.0 percent to a 32 percent increase. Although this description is insufficient to confirm evoked potential sex differences, it does suggest that the reports of such differences in amplitude have some merit and deserve further consideration. Because of its retest variability, amplitude has received less attention than latency.

Age-related variations in amplitude and intensity have also been reported. Hecox and Galambos[24] found that wave V latency was prolonged at birth and that maturation to adult response time occurred primarily by 12 months. Their infant data show latency as a function of age, making it clear that the clinician must take into account the neural maturation of the patient. In fact, since wave V latencies may be no earlier at suprathreshold than 8 to 9 msec in the first few weeks of life, including premature birth, response acquisition requires a longer dwell time (up to 20 msec) than the normally recommended gate of 10 msec for brain stem responses.

The data of Mokotoff and coworkers[7] included premature infants and demonstrated that response latency is a function of gestational age. The reasons for the delay are not fully established, though the data suggest normal changes in myelin as well as maturation of the auditory system. Galambos has also indicated that absorption of mesenchime in the neonate is slow and this material provides a conductive block to the sound.[24] The delay is not a simple conductive disorder, since central conduction times are also prolonged in comparison to normal subjects. Amplitude may be greater in infants because it is easier to establish low electrode resistance, and the connecting tissues are more efficient conductors. In general, wave V responses are large in amplitude, making them highly visible and reliable for interpretation.[23] In adults, there is a tendency for latency to increase with age greater than 50.

In our own review of central conduction time in 14 females age 60 to 74 years, with essentially normal hearing (threshold 25 dB to 40 dB hearing level [HL] at 4000 and 8000 Hz), there was no significant difference in wave V latency in comparison with younger adults. A male group of 10 ears with essentially normal audiological responses presented a mean wave V latency 0.3 msec greater than that of young normal subjects, with prolongation spread over the entire series of waves and not confined to upper or lower brain stem responses. The range of these men for wave I to wave V conduction time was greater than for younger men, since two subjects had latencies well within normal limits. These results do not prove a latency shift in the aging population, but they do suggest the need to investigate average latency in the geriatric population. Until further documentation is available, we assume that aging affects both ears symmetrically in auditory conduction, so that geriatric patients at the upper limits of normal range of latency serve as their own control. More emphasis should be placed on interaural differences in this instance than on statistically normal wave V latency with these patients.

Stockard and coworkers[23] described variations in response secondary to hypothermia, in which reduced body temperature was found to prolong conduction time slightly. Although such patients are infrequently seen, they may be found among drug overdose and comatose subjects. For this reason clinicians should consider this factor in the analysis of potential hypothermia subjects, even though there is insufficient data to predict latency in a known hypothermic patient. Significant temperature-related effects may occur in the presence of demyelinating disease. A neurological history of multiple sclerosis patients often reveals exacerbation of symp-

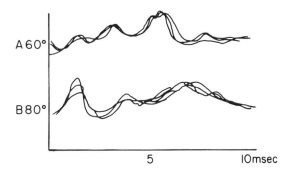

Figure 3-11. Responses for a 28-year-old female with multiple sclerosis. Condition A at 60°F room temperature approaches normal with good retest. Condition B at 80°F suggests a decrease in retest. The figure includes three binaural averages for both conditions.

toms when the patient is hot and perspiring but amelioration of symptoms with cooling. We performed BERA on a patient with multiple sclerosis at 60°F and then at 80°F with the patient in thermal blankets and complaining of overheating. The patient's body temperature was not obtained, since this was only an attempt to determine whether BERA could document this patient's complaint. As demonstrated in Figure 3-11, the wave morphology approached normal under cool conditions but showed markedly poor retest with the patient complaining of being uncomfortably warm.

Since response acquisition is the result of appropriate instrumentation and technique, it is important to leave the protocol flexible and in the hands of a skilled and insightful clinician. "Cookbook" approaches are helpful, but following rigid procedures will result in insufficient response data, particularly when abnormal auditory systems are being evaluated. When the clinician encounters unusual responses, he must be sufficiently sophisticated to manipulate stimulus variables to try to confirm the nature of the auditory abnormality and to rule out error in instrumentation.

Response Interpretation

Response interpretation primarily involves analysis of latency and amplitude. Although both vary with stimulus sensation level, latency is a highly retestable sequence, but amplitude is markedly less so. For most clinical applications, the emphasis is on the latency of the waves. Since stimulus characteristics affect latency, each laboratory needs to establish its own normative data. At suprathreshold level, wave V latency is on the order of 5 to 6 msec, with each preceding wave about 1 msec earlier. However, there is a very small range for normal adult response to a given signal, on the order of 0.2 msec for most commonly used stimuli. The exceptions for sex and age have already been described. To interpret the data with such precision, the clinician must define the normal range for his own technique and stimulus.

How does one report his results? First, the test interpretation is shaped by the purpose of the procedure. If threshold assessment is the object, wave V latency increases are monitored as intensity is decreased. At some intensity level, the latency for wave V will be approximately 8 to 9 msec, with repeatability. With a 10 dB decrease beyond this, there will be no recordable, retestable bump in the averaged EEG. Threshold for wave V is commonly defined as the lowest intensity at which the response is visible in the recording. This technique will allow a threshold search as well as a plot of latency versus intensity. For high-frequency sounds, the threshold for wave V is highly retestable under good conditions and is approximately 10 dB above the voluntary threshold for perception of the signal in normal-hearing adults. It is important to remember that signals approaching 1000 Hz produce poorer retest results, with responses visible only at approximately 30 dB above threshold by routine audiometry. Interpretation of BERA thresholds should incorporate not only comment on the actual threshold of the response but also awareness of the relationship of its significance in terms of a normal response.

Site-of-lesion analysis is generally attempted for suprathreshold averages and should consist of comparison of interwave latencies I to V. Although the label of central conduction may not be altogether technically accurate for the wave I to wave V travel time, it is a useful term in describing results. Since this index looks at responses above threshold in the cochlea, in effect it eliminates so-called delay resulting from inner ear pathology. If central conduction time is not considered, interpretation of delay in the latency of wave V must include a possible delay in brain stem conduction, an elevated threshold of response in the cochlea, or an attenuation in the form of middle ear disease. In such situations wave V responses can be interpreted only in the face of other information about the auditory system. For example, a clinician testing a comatose patient with head injuries and with no other information available may obtain a wave V at 7 msec from both sides at 85 peSPL. How should he interpret such responses? Could they represent cochlear deficit? The patient could have experienced considerable vascular distress or may have a prior history of sensorineural loss. Do they represent a massive brain stem lesion? Too little is known at this point to make a definite interpretation. The clinician should then look for central conduction time. If he finds wave I at 3.8 msec in both ears, he is now able to report normal central conduction time and can begin to suspect that the patient's response is the result of attenuation at the middle ear or cochlea. He can further enhance his interpretation with latency-intensity functions and bone-conduction responses. Conversely, suppose this comatose patient presents a normal latency of wave I in both ears. Since wave I to wave V conduction is prolonged, the clinician may now look to the auditory nerve and brain stem for the problem. He may even find that by looking at wave I to wave II, wave II to wave III, and each successive interval he may be able to speculate more precisely about the level of the auditory breakdown. Although central conduction time or some variant of this index is not universally reported, several authors have found it a sensitive tool.[6,11,14]

Straightforward comparison of absolute wave V latency against mean and range for wave V is also sensitive though less reflective of site of auditory breakdown. With absolute latency comparisons, the examiner must be careful to take into account the possibility of asymmetrical peripheral loss resulting in differences in latency between ears. Since wave V latency decreases as suprathreshold stimulus intensity increases, the examiner must take the latency intensity function under consideration. For example, a subject may present a voluntary threshold for the click stimulus that is 50 dB poorer in the impaired ear than in the opposite ear. The procedure was run at 70 dB above the good ear threshold so that the response reflected abnormal latency from the good side but with only a 20-dB sensation level (SL) to the impaired ear, and wave V was delayed by comparison. Clearly this test is biased by differences in the stimulation sensation level, and any comparison of absolute latency of wave V will reflect it. The impaired ear response could wrongly be interpreted as a central delay when it is in fact only an averaged response at a low sensation level. If the patient voluntary or BERA threshold suggests severe reduction in sensitivity, absolute latency data comparisons cannot be made without other information. Alternatives include (1) assessment of latency-intensity functions to compare ears at an equal sensation level about wave V threshold, (2) increase in stimulus intensity (if possible) to yield a wave V at its earliest possible latency in that ear, and (3) aborting the procedure in favor of other special tests that can be interpreted even with severe loss present. With caution, analysis of latency of wave V is a useful index for interpreting BERA responses.

Interaural comparisons are also useful in response analysis. Since variations related to sex, age, and other factors should have a symmetrical effect, any difference between ears is thought to suggest breakdown in the auditory pathways on the slower side. Selters and Brackmann[6] have found this to be a sensitive comparison for these subjects. In our own experience, interaural comparison of central conduction time from waves I to V is an excellent tool for reducing the rate of misinterpretation, primarily because it eliminates the bias in difference in peripheral sensitivity.

Latency-intensity functions also provide assistance in analysis of the site of the lesion. Separation of cochlear deficit from conductive loss can be enhanced by consideration of latency-intensity changes.[5,24] If the latency of wave V is plotted as a function of intensity, the normal subject will yield a curve ranging about 3 msec from threshold to about 50 dB SL. The conductive loss will yield a function parallel to the normal, but the conductive lesion will be displaced by the amount of the loss. In cochlear lesions the curve steepens, so that less intensity increase is needed to achieve the earliest latency of wave V. We have observed this phenomenon only when there is high-frequency hearing loss, thus often excluding "early" Meniere's disease. In 73 ears assessed by latency functions with clinical diagnosis of cochlear disorder, primarily Meniere's disease, the mean threshold for the click response was 53.3 peSPL (range 35 to 75 dB); that is, 86.3 percent were found to have a steep latency-intensity function, whereas 13.7 percent had displaced, but otherwise normal curves. Although in our series a steep latency-intensity function was seen only in cochlear pathology conditions, not all cochlear ears had steep functions. Some patients with sensorineural loss exhibit normal latency-intensity functions, possibly reflecting differences related to types of cochlear disorder. Latency-intensity functions help to document the site of the lesion, but care must be taken to support interpretation by other techniques such as impedance audiometry.

In comparison to the relatively precise application of latency interpretation, close amplitude evaluations are more difficult to make. This is so because of the relative amplitude of the various waves among normal subjects, and retest amplitudes vary considerably more than retest latencies. Interpolation of absolute amplitude is also more difficult, since baselines float and retest produces variation; however, such gross variations as noted by Stockard and Rossiter[8] are clinically useful observations. There are patients whose wave I amplitude will be markedly large— for example, in comparison to normal range and other responses in that ear. In our experience, morphological variants of a gross nature are often followed by deterioration in the remaining waves. A normal variation is an increase in wave V response amplitude of about 75 per cent with binaural stimulation if the signal intensity if above threshold bilaterally. There is some suggestion that failure to achieve such amplitude increase with binaural stimulation represents abnormality in the upper brain stem. Figure 3–12 demonstrates this relatively subtle abnormality in a subject with multiple sclerosis. Explanations for such changes are only speculative but theoretically may reflect the breakdown of monitoring or feedback in the presence of a massive disorder of the auditory pathways. Gross variations in amplitude help document abnormality even though we do not understand fully the mechanisms involved. As technique is improved, closer monitoring of amplitude range should sharpen the clinical interpretation of BERA responses.

In summary, response analysis consists of consideration of latency and amplitude. Because of high reliability, latency relations can be inspected closely for wave V latency, wave-to-wave conduction times, and

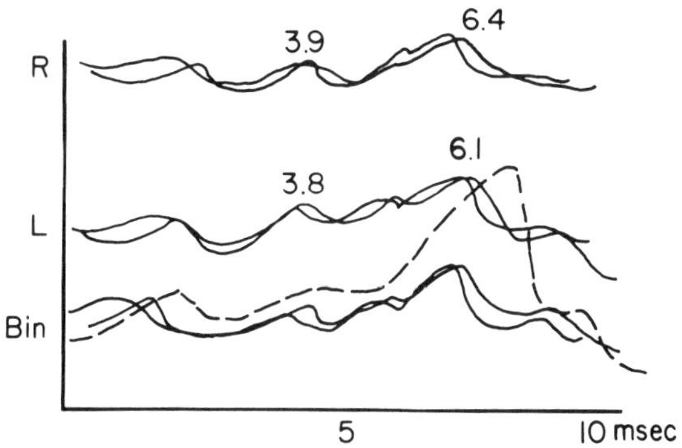

Figure 3-12. Responses from a patient with multiple sclerosis. Right and left ear responses show slight prolongation at waves III to V. Binaural test does not result in the normal amplitude increase (represented by the dotted line). Sample 1K, 8 pps, 85 dB peSPL, 0.1 msec (filtered click).

interaural differences in latency. Gross variations from normal in amplitude should also be noted.

RESPONSE REPORTING

Since the clinician must be prepared to share test results with colleagues in a variety of disciplines, it is important to make the interpretation relevant to the patient's overall diagnostic and rehabilitative program. The report should compare the brain stem responses to predicted behavioral thresholds, with care to point out the critical limitations of this technique. The threshold responses should be reported for wave V but not in any way as representing the same auditory capacity indicated by volunteered thresholds for pure tones. Likewise, the site-of-lesion report should be as specific to point of breakdown as reasonable with the caveat that each wave in the sequence does not directly reflect a specific nucleus. The responses will provide evidence sometimes consistent with conductive disorder, or other instances with cochlear pathology, eighth nerve or low brain stem breakdown, and so on. It is possible to attempt to be more specific in assigning the site of lesion than present data will permit. The wise clinician will also avoid any attempt at diagnosis of the abnormality, since any response variation may be caused by one of several pathological conditions. One patient complaining of bilateral tinnitus was referred after an apparent delay in wave V was thought to represent a bilateral eighth nerve lesion. A subsequent work-up revealed severe high-frequency sensorineural loss bilaterally with normal central conduction on BERA at a higher intensity than in the earlier test. A myelogram was performed with no evidence of a space-occupying lesion. Special tests were otherwise consistent with a cochlear pathological condition bilaterally (by history, noise-induced loss).

The test report should also be helpful in providing some information about conditions, since there is no standard protocol for testing. Other clinicians need to know the test conditions, including the type of stimulus, the repetition rate, the number of samples per average, the stimulus intensity, the retest reliability of the response, whether the patient is sedated or awake, and the basis for defining abnormal response. Only in this manner can consideration to repeating or documenting results be given, until such time as some of these variables are specified in a commonly accepted protocol.

In summary, attempting to define the kind of disease with BERA of the lesion is a serious abuse of the test. In addition, interpretation of BERA without any other data whether subjective or in the form of other procedures such as routine audiometry or impedance audiometry or whatever protocol is possible is an unwarranted gamble. Seldom are all tests except BERA precluded. Interpreting responses must be based on the framework of documentation by other audiological procedures, BERA retest, and other clinical information, including the patient's history.

CALIBRATION TECHNIQUE

The clinician should monitor equipment output as part of routine maintenance. Much of the maintenance has to do with verifying timer characteristics, averager performance, and other technical considerations that can be monitored by the manufacturer or by someone trained in computer electronics. The stimulus, however, should be monitored at the test site for the same reasons that a standard audiometer requires a calibration check. Determining sound pressure level (SPL) output is not as straightforward as a routine audiometer output check, because the stimuli are brief in duration. If a sound level meter with impulse capture is available, output at the transducer can be observed. Alternatively peSPL can be determined by displaying the signal on an oscilloscope and noting the peak-to-peak amplitude. With the same set-up, a known pure tone is driven through the transducer (generally at the resonant frequency of the earphone) and adjusted to provide the same peak-to-peak amplitude as the test stimulus on the oscilloscope. The SPL required to match amplitude as indicated at the SPL meter is the peak equivalent SPL of the stimulus. Either of these techniques will provide a reference for monitoring output, since there is minimal information standardizing specification of click or brief tone intensity. In addition, biological calibration between laboratory checks will help to monitor changes in output. Normal threshold for click can be established with a normal "jury" of 5 or 10 subjects as used in our clinic to provide a basis for biological calibration.

Another consideration in calibration is monitoring for any changes in frequency response. Stimulus shape should be defined when new equipment is received. If periodic comparisons are to reveal a significant documentation change, the clinician must monitor not only the electrical impulse but also the acoustical form of the signal through the transducer to be used in the clinic. Otherwise important considerations such as rise time and peak stimulus frequency will not be adequately included in interpretation of the section of the auditory system under test. Generator or transducer malfunction can be rarely be ''heard'' even by the so-called trained listener. For this reason acoustical output should be included as part of the calibration procedure.

REVIEW OF TEST TECHNIQUE

The following sections are a review with emphasis on suggestions of test protocol, or a kind of ''game plan.'' It is important to stress that the protocol must be flexible for the insightful clinician to capture as much information as possible about the auditory system of the individual. At the same time, the procedure is somewhat determined by the characteristics of the equipment being used for evoking the potentials.

The plan is determined by the nature of the primary information being sought, roughly grouped as either threshold search or site-of-lesion test. If the purpose of the test is to obtain thresholds, the following guidelines are a good model to follow, although they are not a hard-and-fast plan. (It assumes that the clinician has already obtained normative data with his equipment.)

Provide a quiet, relaxing setting with a couch or bed for supine testing. Before attempting to obtain a suitable test state, the electrodes should be fixed. If a child is to nap, electrodes should be fixed with the electrode wires out of reach before he relaxes, as there is no need to arouse or antagonize him after he settles down. It also helps to feed the child, just prior to testing, and to provide him with a pillow or favorite blanket or anything else to suggest naptime. For some reason, perhaps boredom, a large number of subjects drowse or sleep during testing even though the first several averages may look noisy. For this reason we nearly always anticipate patient cooperation without the use of drugs. By affixing the electrodes immediately and attempting to acquire a response, we are generally able to achieve recordable responses. With infants it is sometimes necessary to introduce the signal with a hand-held earphone or mounted speaker until deep sleep is achieved.

If the aforementioned techniques do not satisfactorily prepare the patient and a repeatable wave cannot be measured, an artifact must be suspected. Although an absence of repeatable waves in an awake patient may reflect auditory problems, retest in a state of sleep will be necessary to validate the response. The supervising physician will determine the method of sedation based on patient age and health. With some subjects, such as very young or multiply handicapped patients, administration of general anesthesia to produce light sleep may be considered safer than the use of sedatives and has the further advantage of direct medical surpervision. Since general anesthesia is usually administered in a hospital, the expense and potential risk should be balanced against the need for BERA. Generally, subjecting a child to medication would be contraindicated if auditory behavior could be observed and retested in the sound field. However, since BERA is an important technique in early identification of hearing loss, special procedures such as sedation may be warranted in otherwise difficult cases.

As an example, a Korean orphan aged 2.5 years came to the United States to be adopted by a military family. Only the adopting mother could control or relate to the child without a fear response from him. She suspected deafness as a complicating factor in his failure to communicate. The child also exhibited behavior suggestive of cultural shock and withdrawal, and as he had already experienced several temporary care settings, the team working with the family wanted to rule out hysterical deafness. This child spoke no Korean or English but did reportedly "chatter" while playing. Because of his shyness and withdrawal he alternated between a passive state and sobbing during testing, so that two different hearing clinics were unable to determine with any certainty the degree of hearing loss. Impedance audiometry failed to provide an estimate of the loss because of the child's constant sobbing during repeated tests. In view of the patient's history, the otologist ordered polytomography, a precedure requiring anesthesia for most children less than 7 years of age. While the child was anesthetized, we conducted BERA and impedance audiometry. Tympanometry suggested slight negative pressure with absent reflexes bilaterally. No response was obtained for BERA at maximum intensity. Based on two tests the patient was thought to have a severe auditory disorder. An external canal electrode was positioned next to the tympanic membrane but no N_1 response or action potential was observed, suggesting a severe peripheral deficit. If the child had not been drugged, the absence of response would have been inconclusive, making it the third audiological evaluation unable to rule out or confirm hearing loss. Since the patient was in a monitored sleep state, results were labeled as consistent with a severe bilateral peripheral deficit. Polytomography immediately followed the auditory potential studies and revealed a marked abnormality of both cochleae, providing an unusual instance of immediate substantiation of BERA findings. The child is now in a program for deaf children specially adapted to his unusual language problems. In most cases it is important to continue attempts at traditional audiometry in order to analyze the subject's ability to process whatever sound is provided from the auditory periphery.

Although there are situations in which steps such as the use of anesthesia is warranted, for most patients sedation is sufficient. It is important to provide adequate medical supervision for such cases. For instance, hyperactive patients who cannot be tested by routine methods are quite likely to respond adversely to sedatives such as secobarbital and chloral hydrate. If the activity level increases, it only frustrates the examiner. If there is a shock response, emergency procedures may be necessary to prevent fatality. It is a good practice to suspect the patient's state when BERA results are not subject to reliable retest or are absent. Voluntary sleep represents the optimum patient state for testing. Failing this, medical supervision for drug-induced sleep or anesthesia is in order.

It is possible for an uncooperative subject to obstruct the test without the examiner's knowledge. In a test, for example, the patient can thwart testing by chronic neuromuscular contamination. The example demonstrated in Figure 3-13 was obtained by completing an average with the subject's jaw clenched on demand, with the resulting apparent response abnormality. In our experience wily patients can bias even such objective tests like impedance audiometry and BERA. It may be advisable to obtain sedation for such patients, again with care to ensure medical supervision.

To minimize the duration of the threshold test procedure, begin testing with binaural stimulation at a moderately high intensity, 90 dB peSPL. Using a rapid repetition rate such as 40 pulses per second, binaural stimulation will allow the examiner to scan for wave V threshold, since it has higher visibility with binaural search and persists even at high repetition

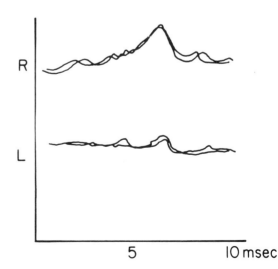

Figure 3-13. Normal subject. Right ear tested during relaxation while subject deliberately clenched teeth for left ear stimulation. Sample 1024 at 8 pps, 60 dB SL (subject threshold), 0.1 msec filtered click.

5   10 msec

rates. The determination of whether both ears are responding can be made by repeating the run stimulating only one side. If the response amplitude is unchanged, probably only one ear is participating; if it drops, both are contributing. For rapid searches, we stimulate binaurally at high repetition rates and relatively small samples (512), with a decrease in intensity until wave V cannot be observed. Near estimated threshold intensity, a large sample (at least 1000) with monaural stimulation at a slower rate (for example, 8 pps) is obtained, varying intensity in 10 dB steps to find the lowest intensity at which wave V can be detected. The same procedure is repeated contralaterally. Reproducibility is verified on retest, then, if possible, stimulus frequency characteristics are altered and the procedure is repeated.

For site-of-lesion testing, the technique must be modified. Best results are obtained with a slow repetition rate, generally less than ten per second with a relatively large sample (1000 or more) and suprathreshold stimulation. In contrast to threshold procedures, patient relaxation is important, but responses can generally be obtained from a quiet patient without requiring a sleep state. Latencies should be recorded, amplitude noted, and the procedure repeated. Latencies should be retestable at no more than 0.1 msec variation for tolerance in reading errors. If the runs do not overlap in latency, the responses cannot be considered reliable. The trouble-shooting section will suggest some techniques when retest results are poor. Some possibilities are poor test evnironment (including patient state), equipment artifact, or an active disease process such as multiple sclerosis. Generally, two trials are sufficient to prove retest, and the examiner can proceed directly to the contralateral ear. If the response appears abnormal it is wise to obtain an average under the same conditions but complete attenuation of the signal. A null or straight-line recording should result, indicating that the bumps in the preceding average reflected auditory response.

Starting with the better side in asymmetrical losses will help the examiner to assess a patient's response pattern for better comparison with the off-side response. If beginning the data collection at 90 peSPL does not provide a normal sequence, the intensity should be increased. As a rule, pure tone audiometry precedes site-of-lesion testing in our clinic. It helps to obtain threshold for the BERA stimulus also. When thresholds are available, intensity for testing can be chosen with little loss of test time. If voluntary threshold is known, the absence of wave V is interpreted more reliably, although the relationship between audibility of the stimulus and number of responders to evoke a synchronous discharge is unknown. In general, when testing at levels known to be suprathreshold, a no-response average should be documented by ruling out equipment errors such as improper input to the preamplifier or operator failure to activate the earphone.

Normal subject responses under the suggested test conditions should provide a highly retestable latency if a somewhat variable amplitude. Using latency data from other laboratories is not advisable because of the variation in available stimuli, preamplifier, and filter characteristics, among other factors. It is far better for the clinician to acquire his own normative values. Absolute range of latency in response to suprathreshold high-frequency signals is low, so that a small group of normal responses will provide a basis for determining the latency range. Once normal responses can be easily identified and repeated, data interpretation can be attempted.

Once patient state is adequate for testing, the variables should be selected to evoke a response that is as easily detected as possible. With these general considerations, the procedure for site-of-lesion testing becomes a checklist.

1. *Appropriate intensity.* Increase intensity to increase detectability of waves.

2. *Set repetition rate.* Increase to eliminate or decrease all wave V, but decrease to enhance earlier waves.

3. *Determine size of sample.* Increase to eliminate noise; decrease if time is a consideration.

4. *Set dwell time.* Ten milliseconds is sufficient for normal adults but a 20 msec sweep time may be necessary to see brain stem responses in young patients and in abnormal brain stems.

5. *Vary amplitude amplification.* Set amplification of the baseline as high as possible without saturating the preamplifier.

6. *Set preamplifier filters to the best compromise of elimination of noise without clipping the response.* For many commercial systems 3000 Hz is the upper end of the clinically useful frequencies, whereas 20 to 150 Hz may be selected as the low pass, depending on equipment, external noise, and desired response characteristics.

7. *Choose ear to be stimulated.* Begin with better ear, if known. Binaural testing should also be considered, since it can save time in some situations and provide significant findings in site-of-lesion analysis in others.

8. *Set artifact rejection rate for reasonable response acquisition.* This is determined by the nature of the rejection system in the equipment. Once the variables are appropriately selected, the clinician is ready to obtain the auditory brain stem responses.

TROUBLESHOOTING

The following outline includes some of the problems encountered clinically in BSER measurement. It is by no means exhaustive, but includes common problems that can be anticipated in clinical settings.

1. A major source of recording error is at the connection of the electrode to the patient. If the average is noisy, recheck the electrode resistances. Resistances may vary during testing, particularly with paste-and-tape as opposed to collodion application. Rebalancing them to less than 5000 ohms will reduce noise. If background noise is not reduced after reapplication, the electrodes should be tested for failure or simply replaced, since the problem may be on the electrode connector to the preamplifier.

2. Occasionally electrode-to-skin contact will be adequate, but there will be an electrical transmission barrier, for example, a steel prosthesis or some types of indwelling shunt. Patient history or prior radiological data will allow the clinician to identify such contaminants. Electrode placement must be varied, or in some cases even recording with the contralateral side as the reference site is a possibility if the clinician is careful to interpret the response with this bias in mind.

3. Large artifacts may represent implants such as a pacemaker. (In such cases extra care to ground the patient is important.) Since these artifacts are large and not time-locked to the stimulus, it may be possible to acquire a response by eliminating artifact reject. A small sample, for instance 512 stimuli, may contain less artifact bias than the normal sweep. If such averages yield unusual responses, it is not possible to make a valid interpretation. The artifact must be eliminated. If this is not possible, the procedure should be terminated in favor of other techniques.

4. Electrical line noise is a common artifact. The test setting should provide a common ground and a proper grounding connection with care to eliminate ground loops. Experimenting with different power plugs within reach may uncover a quieter line, isolated from other electrical noise. Although routine administration should provide shielding against chronic electrical interference, it is not so straightforward in the operating room or intensive care unit. Sampling different power outlets with a grounded connection in the area may produce an isolated power source.

Excessive 60 Hz noise may also reflect an unused input not shorted to ground or an "open" electrode. Making sure that the preamplifier connectors are properly in line and that the electrodes are in good contact will eliminate one source. Straightening power cables and electrode wires will eliminate another cause of such noise. Unplugging unnecessary equipment may also remove error. Fluorescent lights should be turned off, since they are often a noise source.

5. Radiofrequency noise can create a large artifact and is sometimes difficult to eliminate. Trial-and-error repositioning of the equipment and the patient will generally lower this artifact level to adequate quiet. Raising the low-frequency preamplifier cut may also help. In some situations cable and room shielding are necessary.

6. Unrepeatable wave forms can cause a false impression of abnormal-

ity. Before the clinician blames an abnormal or absent response on the patient's auditory response, technical errors (including electrode failure as described earlier) should be considered.

a. Although timer failure is not common, it is possible for the timer to become asynchronous, so that stimuli will be heard in cadence or code. Depending on the nature of the failure, the result can provide bizarre and unrepeatable responses. The patient or the clinician can often detect this problem by listening for cadence or beats.

b. Verify acoustical stimulation to the ear under test by listening to the earphones to rule out equipment failure or improper procedure choice.

c. Recheck electrode resistance.

d. Attempt repetition of the pattern, since the confirmation of abnormality is its reproducibility. It should be noted that some lesions are not static and will not be subject to retest.

e. Sound intensity should be varied to determine whether the abnormal responses are in fact auditory in origin. Both amplitude and latency should change with variation in intensity. If the abnormality is gross enough to make it difficult to identify and label the auditory responses, increasing the repetition rate significantly should diminish all other auditory responses, and the persisting bump can be suspected as wave V.

f. Repeat the average with a silent run but with all other variables held constant. If the response was auditory in origin it will disappear. Anything remaining is an equipment or ground problem, typically 60 Hz noise.

g. Consider potential patient artifacts from major problems such as noisy EEG (obscuring acoustic responses) to such problems as collapsing canals or other conduction impairment reducing signal intensity to the inner ear.

h. If an abnormality—especially no response—persists, the examiner should immediately retest a known normal subject under the same conditions to prove the equipment. (This check, if successful, may be followed by patient retest.) This alternative is sometimes the only accessible double check and is important even if somewhat time consuming.

If the response is variable on retest, a quiet run is virtually straight, and other artifacts have been eliminated, the nature of the lesion can be assumed to be a factor. The clinician can help document patient variability by repeating the procedure with the subject under sedation to rule out myogenic or other patient artifact. It is clinically useful information to demonstrate patient response variation.

In summary, trouble-shooting should include a methodical check on manipulation of the instrumentation and proper patient management. Regular recalibration and periodic monitoring of a known normal subject and a daily check of earphone voluntary threshold should be routine and are as important as standard "biological calibration of the audiometer."

REFERENCES

1. Davis, H.: Principles of electric response audiometry. *Ann Otol Rhinol Laryngol* 85 (Suppl. 28): 1976.
2. Skinner, P. H.: Electroencephalic response audiometry. *In* Katz, J., (ed.): *Handbook of Clinical Audiology,* 2nd ed., pp. 311–327. Baltimore, Williams & Wilkins Co., 1978.
3. Jewett, D. L., Romano, M. N., and Williston, J. S.: Human auditory evoked potentials: Possible brainstem components detected on the scalp. Science 167:1517–1518, 1970.
4. Coats, A., and Martin, J.: Human auditory nerve action potentials and brainstem evoked responses: effects of audiogram shape and lesion location. Arch Otolaryngol 103:605–623, 1977.
5. Jerger, J., Mauldin, L., Anthony, L.: Brain-stem evoked response audiometry. Audiol Hear Educ 4:17, 1978.
6. Selters, W. A. and Brackmann, D. E.: Acoustic tumor detection with brainstem electric response audiometry. Arch Otolaryngol 103:181–187, 1977.
7. Mokotoff, B., Schulmann-Galambos, C., and Galambos, R.: Brainstem auditory evoked responses in children. Arch Otolaryngol 103:38–43, 1977.
8. Stockard, J. J., and Rossiter, V. S.: Clinical and pathologic correlates of brainstem auditory response abnormalities. Neurology 27:316–325, 1977.
9. Starr, A., and Hamilton, A. F.: Correlation between confirmed sites of neurological lesions and abnormalities of far-field auditory brainstem response. Electroencephalogr Clin Neurophysiol 41:595–608, 1976.
10. Clemis, J. D., and McGee, T.: Brainstem electric response audiometry in the differential diagnosis of acoustic tumors. Laryngoscope 89:31–42, 1979.
11. Glasscock, M. E., Jackson, C. G., Josey, A. F., Dickens, J. R. E., and Wiet, R.: Brainstem evoked response audiometry in a clinical practice. Laryngoscope 89:1021–1035, 1979.
12. Goff, W. R., Williamson, P. D., van Gilder, J. C. et. al.: Neural origins of long latency evoked potentials recorded from the depth and cortical surface of the brain in man. Brussels, Proceedings of the International Symposium on Cerebral Evoked Potentials in Man, 1979.
13. Berlin, C. I., and Dobie, R. A.: Electrophysiological measures of auditory function via electrocochleography and brainstem evoked responses. *In* Rintelmann, W. F. (ed.): *Hearing Assessment.* Baltimore, University Park Press, 1979.
14. Starr, A., and Achor J.: Auditory Brainstem Response in Neurological Disease. Arch Neurol 32:761–768, 1975.
15. Stockard, J. J., and Jones, T. A.: Central nervous system drugs and the brainstem evoked response. Electroencephalogr Clin Neurophysiol 43:550, 1977.
16. Squires, K. C., Chu, N., and Starr, A.: Acute effects of alcohol on auditory brainstem potentials in man. Science 201:174–176, 1978.
17. Fria, T. J., and Sabo, D. L.: The use of brainstem auditory electric responses in children: practical considerations. Hear Aid J March:30–32, 1979.
18. Eggermont, J. J., Odenthal, D. W., Schmidt, P. H., and Spoor, A.: Electrocochleography: basic principles and clinical applications. Acta Otolaryngol 316:1–84, 1979.
19. Weber, B. A., and Fujikawa, S. M.: Brainstem evoked response (BER) audiometry at various stimulus presentation rates. J Am Audiol Soc 3:59, 1977.
20. Thornton, A. R. D., and Coleman, M. J.: The adaptation of cochlear and brainstem auditory evoked potentials in humans. Electroencephalogr Clin Neurophysiol 39:399–406, 1975.

21. Daly, D. R., Rosen, R. T., Aung, M. U., and Daly D. D.: Early evoked potential in patients with acoustic neuroma. Electroencephalogr Clin Neurophysiol 43:151–159, 1977.
22. Sanders, J. W., Josey, A. F., Glasscock, M.: Audiologic evaluation in cochlear and eighth nerve disorders. Arch Otolaryngol 100:283–289, 1974.
23. Stockard, J. J., Stockard, J. G., and Sharbrough, F. W.: Nonpathological factors influencing brainstem auditory evoked potentials. Am J EEG Technol 18:177–209, 1978.
24. Hecox, K., and Galambos, R.: Brainstem auditory evoked responses in human infants and adults. Arch Otolaryngol 99:30–33, 1974.

Chapter Four

CLINICAL APPLICATIONS OF BERA

INTRODUCTION

Auditory evoked potentials were identified in the human electro encephalogram (EEG) by Davis in 1939.[1] The application of biological averaging concepts and the development of averaging computer technology in 1961 have propelled this laboratory technique into the mainstream of clinical audiology and neurotology. As equipment is updated and experience is expanded, specialized areas of application continue to be proposed. It is the clinical usefulness of this technique to which this chapter is directed.

BASIC INFORMATION

Myriad auditory electric responses have been described and monitored at varying latencies from their stimulated initiation. Responses are generally grouped, based on their individual latencies, into (1) slow, cortical responses—50 to 60 msec, (2) middle responses—12 to 50 msec, and (3) fast responses—occurring within the first 10 msec. It is the fast responses, including those from the cochlear and brain stem pathways, that are clinically the most useful and that comprise the measured activity of brain stem electric response and audiometry (BERA).

Auditory electric brain stem responses represent far-field reflections of electrical events occurring within the auditory pathway from the cochlear end-organ as they proceed through brain stem pathways to the auditory cortex. Since electrodes are not in direct contact with the neurophysiological electrical generators themselves, "far field" recording is necessary. By convention,[2,3] the recording is represented by a series of waves, each identified by a Roman numeral. Wave I has been accepted as representing the eighth nerve action potential. All subsequent waves, however, must realistically be assumed to represent the combined electrical input of multiple contributory centers throughout the auditory pathway. Several investigators have suggested that each wave may be the product of a specific neural generator.[4-7] Wave II is thought to be generated by the cochlear nuclei, wave III by the superior olivary complex, wave IV within

77

the lateral lemniscus, and wave V by the inferior colliculus. Waves VI and VII represent unknown centers. Although probably a neurophysiological oversimplification, the data of Starr and Hamilton[4] suggest this scheme is clinically useful, and it is within this context that we shall operate.

Wave V has been established as the most stable and is the most clinically useful. Wave V latency and its relation to other wave forms and to the stimulus compose the primary data evaluated by BERA. A more detailed analysis of the neurophysiological and bioacoustical principles of recording as they relate to the generation and interpretation of data can be found in Chapter 3.

Wave V latency and the BERA audiogram are determined by stimulus parameters, cochlear function, and neural transmission along both the eighth nerve and the brain stem auditory pathways.[8] The response is objective, with variations in states of arousal, awareness, or attention being irrelevant. We have at our disposal, then, an objective method for the direct evaluation of auditory function from the cochlear end-organ up to and including the auditory centers of the brain stem. The ability to localize auditory pathology to the cochlea, the eighth nerve, or the central transmission pathways remarkably expands the cochlear versus retro-cochlear behavioral limitation. Each anatomical contributor to the auditory response can be considered separately, giving "site-of-lesion" testing its purest definition.

Site-of-lesion determination can be expanded indirectly to include those forms of pathological processes that impose functional abnormalities in auditory function as an extrinsic force or perhaps as a more diffuse process. Specifically, lesions of the cerebellopontine angle, the eighth nerve, or the temporal bone often will produce effects altering normal auditory function. Objective documentation of brain stem pathology in the form of demyelinating disease, neoplasia, or vascular embarrassment can be made as a result of their effects on brain stem auditory pathways.

In addition to the classic site-of-lesion testing so applicable to the clinical practice of neurotology,[9–11] the utility of BERA to site-of-lesion determination within the field of neurology has been established.[5,12] BERA is also an objective evaluator of auditory function in the assessment of peripheral threshold sensitivity.[13–15] Being more sensitive and objective in the evaluation of site of lesion and peripheral system functional integrity, BERA emerges a repeatable and reliable reinforcement of standard behavioral audiology protocols.

BERA neither replaces the standard site-of-lesion formats nor does it render behavioral audiometry obsolete. Rather, it serves an adjunctive role as an integral part of the diagnostic plan individually formulated to evaluate the complaint of the neurotological patient.

NEUROTOLOGICAL EVALUATION

When BERA is used as part of a neurotological evaluation site-of-lesion determination, differentiating cochlear from retrocochlear disease, including acoustic tumor, is its most crucial diagnostic function. The presence or absence of wave V, its latency, and an analysis of central conduction times are the most vital determinants.

The neurotological test battery includes pure tone and speech audiometry, stapedial reflex decay and latency, Olsen modification of the Carhart tone decay test, modified SISI, electronystagmography (ENG), petrous pyramid x-rays, and when indicated, BERA. An increase in diagnostic concern prompted by abnormality in any test in this battery describes, as necessary, the application of computed axial tomography (CAT) scanning, with and without contract enhancement, as well as posterior fossa myelography. A positive CAT scan precludes posterior fossa myelography in the vast majority of cases. CAT scanning is becoming a more regular part of the routine evaluation of those patients suspected of having retrocochlear disease. Lesions smaller than 1.5 to 2.0 cm often fail to exceed the resolving capabilities of the CAT scanner.[16] To identify these cases, posterior fossa myelography is obtained even when the CAT scan result is negative; however, the battery of tests makes retrocochlear pathology highly suspect.

BERA is 98 per cent accurate in determining surgically confirmed eighth nerve lesions.[11] Consequently, when the neurotological evaluation, including BERA and CAT scan, does not suggest retrocochlear pathology, posterior fossa myelography is generally deferred. Identification of significant vestibular paresis, erosion of an internal auditory canal, or other audiometric inconsistency, despite no abnormality of BERA, mandates posterior fossa myelography, which is still our most reliable indicator of pathology in this area.

As is the case with any test, the clinical utility of BERA is not without limitations. To generate the data of BERA, the stimulus must be presented at levels approximately 50 dB Sound Level (SL) (40 to 50 dB above threshold). Hearing that is poorer than 70 to 80 dB, as may be associated with an acoustic tumor, will exceed the capability of the test and will generate the concept of an "untestable ear." Similarly, retrocochlear lesions other than neurolemmoma seem to generate a higher incidence of "false negative" information that do acoustic tumors when tested using BERA.[1] Thus, there are two major limitations to proposing BERA as the single, definitive site-of-lesion determination. Rather than displace conventional site-of-lesion protocols, BERA must assume its proper perspective as a powerful adjunct to the neurotological evaluation.

In addition to its more substantial contribution to site-of-lesion accuracy, BERA is an effective and objective evaluator of the status of the brain stem. In more specific circumstances, BERA similarly reinforces behavioral techniques in threshold testing. A more detailed description of applicability in these clinical situations follows.

CLINICAL SITUATIONS

Threshold Testing

Problems associated with assessing auditory function in difficult-to-test situations has, for years, stimulated a search for an objective indicator to complement data supplied by behavioral measures. In this regard, auditory evoked potentials have been shown to be invaluable. For threshold determination the most accurate evoked potentials are those measured by E Co G. BERA appears safer, since it requires only surface electrode placement and usually can be performed without significant anesthesia or sedation. Furthermore BERA is superior in generating more diagnostic information. Localization of a lesion to a specific site within the auditory pathway is possible without sacrificing accuracy of threshold determination. Most investigators [7,17-21] document thresholds obtained by BERA to agree within 5 to 15 dB of those confirmed by behavioral measures in normal subjects or when lesions could be reliably assessed.

A point of emphasis must be established. No objective neurophysiological test analysis can replace the information obtained by standard pure tone and speech tests. These are the most reliable determinators of what a patient actually "hears." We must remember that BERA monitors only the functional integrity of the "peripheral system" up to and including the brain stem auditory centers. Cortical integrative function is not evaluated. BERA is, however, a very precise index of the efficiency with which the peripheral auditory organ receives and transmits centrally acoustic energy. What the patient does with this acoustic information can be evaluated only within standard behavioral formats.

Candidates for application of BERA to threshold determination are those cases in which behavioral techniques are not possible. Those situations in which the patient is unable or unwilling to generate a standard audiogram predominate. Infants, young children, the mentally handicapped, and malingerers compose the majority of those who are difficult to test.

There is a growing body of evidence that now confirms hearing loss as contributing to significant learning and speech disability even when these losses are mild or fluctuating. Early identification of this decreased acuity is often easier acknowledged than accomplished. With this in mind, BERA has been applied to newborn infant screening, particularly in high-risk groups.[22]

BERA in newborns and in very young children has been documented as accurate.[22-26] The facility with which BERA is applied in this situation is far superior to the practical problems of respiratory audiometry, heart rate methods, or cribogram and behavioral techniques. BERA has been particularly productive in the high-risk population of neonates admitted to intensive care units (ICUs). The use of ototoxic drugs, oxygenation abnormalities, bilirubin problems, and an otherwise high incidence of associated abnormalities justify screening of auditory function in this population. Schulman-Galambos and Galambos[22] reported an incidence of hearing loss in 2.14 per cent of this high-risk group as opposed to 0 per cent in a similarly tested normal population. Particularly in these high-risk groups, he has recommended routine auditory screening using BERA.

The several case reports with comment that follow are representative of the spectrum of the clinical applicability of BERA in threshold confirmation.

Case 1

G.F. is a 6-week-old infant girl who was the product of a complicated pregnancy. In the first trimester of the pregnancy, the mother contracted severe bilateral pyelonephritis with moderate degrees of renal failure. Sustained levels of high-dose, potentially ototoxic antibiotics were administered. Even so, disease control was poor. On several occasions, termination of the pregnancy was suggested, but the mother declined despite the significant threat posed to her own life.

At 8 months gestation, the pregnancy was terminated by the premature delivery of the 7.7 kg patient. The child's prematurity, low birthweight, hyperbilirubinemia, and exposure to high doses of potentially ototoxic antibiotics clearly placed her at high risk. Indeed we were asked to test her in a neonatal ICU.

Screening auditory tests administered in the ICU failed to demonstrate any consistent response. BERA was easily performed. Results revealed normal thresholds bilaterally and normal auditory function at least to the level of the inferior colliculus.

Comment: The BERA findings in this situation greatly relieved the child's parents who had agonized over each decision made during the mother's pregnancy. They held themselves personally responsible for even the possibility of their child's hearing loss. Continued follow-up to confirm the BERA findings and to permit evaluation of cortical integrative function will be necessary. If a hearing loss had been identified, auditory rehabilitation could have been acknowledged as a major dimension in this high-risk child's future therapeutic direction, one in which audition and language will be even more important than in normal developmental circumstances.

The diagnosis of hearing loss in young children is similarly crucial yet even more problematical. Improved language skills and better psychosocial adjustment are the dividends of early diagnosis and hearing rehabilitation, especially in children less than 1 year of age and specifically no later than 3 years of age. BERA can be a reliable back-up to behavioral formats for this population.

Mentally and physically handicapped children constitute a majority of candidates for BERA evaluation. Inconsistent and confusing behavioral audiometric data resulting from limitations in attention span and an inability to comprehend behavioral techniques very often represent reasons for BERA testing. The objectivity and accuracy of BERA is capable of resolving problems of delayed or incompletely formulated rehabilitative treatment planning, which is often the result of inconclusive and inconsistent behavioral data.

A major problem in evaluating the accuracy of any testing technique applied to this type of situation is verification of data. Results in normal subjects[7,17-21] with behavioral follow-up confirm the accuracy of BERA; however, some question remains as to its efficiency in these very pathological cases. Emphasis must then be appropriately placed upon not any one diagnostic agent but rather a battery of tests as we do in site-of-lesion testing. Behavioral audiometry, impedance measurements, and BERA must be closely linked to responsible follow-up for data verification if and when behavioral techniques afford reliable data, that is, when the child is older. In some circumstances, E Co G may be useful, especially when considering the appropriateness of amplification devices.

Although some studies report variability of evoked potentials in children, particularly during sleep or under sedation,[23-26] follow-up data on these children assessed by BERA has resolved many of these problems. Hume and Cont,[26] in a follow-up study, found 32 of 34 patients correctly diagnosed by BERA. The principal source of error identified in their study was the use of barbiturate sedation, a problem inconsistently acknowledged. Similarly, patients who had experienced encephalitis or meningitis most commonly exhibited diagnostic error. Mokotoff and associates[27] have also shown BERA to be remarkably accurate. They showed that in a majority of cases (76.5 per cent), BERA confirmed the existing clinical impression. A tribute can thereby be generated to behavioral audiometry, and the concept of test battery is reinforced. BERA then serves as a reliable reinforcement of conventional testing, but also provides additional information in localizing lesions, information that may enhance rehabilitation of these problem children.

When an error is generated by BERA, rarely is the audiologist-physician team dangerously misled.[26] The most common error generated by BERA testing is the incorrect diagnosis of a hearing loss, the consequences of which are far less serious than those associated with the false diagnosis of normal hearing in the hearing-impaired child.

Case 2

D.L. is a 3-year-old white male in whom pure tone, sound field, and impedance audiometry suggested thresholds in the 60 to 70 dB range. His mother sought medical attention for him because he was nonverbal. Hearing aids had not improved communication skills appreciably. He has had recurrent otitis media and has been hospitalized twice with pneumonia.

BERA data were recorded following insertion of ventilation tubes under general anesthesia (Fig. 4-1). On the left, waves I and II were present. Only wave I was identified on the right. Total dysynchrony and obliteration of subsequent wave forms indicated severe auditory brain stem dysfunction. Thresholds were confirmed at 60 dB bilaterally.

Comment: This child represents an unusual problem of brain stem auditory pathway pathology, the etiology of which is unknown. Amplification is of little use to him, so appropriate education and rehabilitative measures were prescribed. Wave I (compound action potential) is not always as clearly defined as it is in this child.[13] When wave I is less discernible, a battery of tests, including E Coch G, should be employed before therapeutic recommenda-

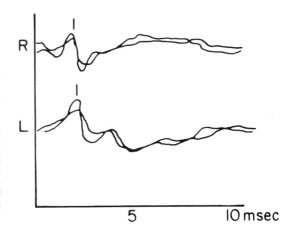

Figure 4-1. BERA, case 2, D.L. Bilateral retrocochlear pathology, specifically brain stem dysfunction. Note wave I preservation. See text for description. (BERA procedural recording standards apply to this tracing as well as all subsequent recordings illustrated in this chapter: 0.1 = msec click duration delivered at 40 to 60 dB SL re threshold unless otherwise indicated; repetition rate of eight per second; 50-Hz lower and 3000-Hz upper filters.

tions can be made. In this case, however, E Coch G would add nothing to diagnosis or rehabilitative strategy.

Case 3

R.K. is a 12-year-old white male who was left severely psychomentally retarded as a sequela of encephalitis following vaccination for measles in early childhood. Chronic infectious ear disease made the control of an underlying seizure disorder increasingly difficult. Chronic otitis media with cholesteatoma in the right ear indicated surgical intervention. As a result of his severe mental retardation, behavioral audiometry was impossible. The child's mother and some nurses were able to communicate with him, even if on a primitive level. In fear of compromising this level of communication, we did not want to risk surgery on an only hearing ear. Auditory information about the left ear was crucial.

BERA was performed under sedation and results confirmed normal thresholds bilaterally. Consequently, surgery was performed safely and confidently. A much different surgical approach would have been necessary had the operated ear been, as well, an only hearing ear.

BERA is especially useful in threshold determination in situations in which accurate behavioral evaluation of auditory sensitivity is questionable as a result of the subject's unwillingness to generate a standard audiogram. By 1954, more than 40 behavioral test formats had been described to aid in defining the true level of auditory sensitivity in uncooperative patients.[28] Classically known as malingering tests, these protocols have been remarkably effective in distinguishing organic and functional disorders. Certain test patterns as well as the psychological characteristics of these subjects often leave little doubt that a hearing loss has no organic basis.

Once the diagnosis or suspicion of functional hearing loss has been made clinically by one or more behavioral tests, definition of the patient's true level of auditory ability becomes the objective. Behavioral tests can approximate thresholds in most of these cases; however, they do not satisfactorily measure the absolute or true level of auditory acuity. BERA, as a completely objective indicator of auditory function, not only confirms the existence of a functional hearing loss but also accurately defines the inconsistent patient's auditory thresholds completely without his cooperation and, specifically, despite his unwillingness to generate appropriate responses. Referral for psychiatric evaluation and therapy can be made with greater equanimity with objective test information at hand. McCandless and Lentz[29] report a series of 32 cases in which the usefulness of BERA was established in the determination of thresholds in these uncooperative patients. Again, we can conclude that BERA is an important reinforcement of standard protocols in difficult-to-test situations. Inclusion into the clinician's diagnostic armamentarium is recommended.

Case 4

B.B. is a 15-year-old female who underwent an appendectomy. Enjoying an uneventful recovery and 1 day prior to her discharge (1 week postoperatively) she apparently had an adverse reaction to an intramuscular injection of pain medication and became violent, combative, and irrational. Her mother defined this as a seizure, but two observing nurses would not confirm this. Several hours later, after gaining control, the patient complained of a total (bilateral) loss of hearing. Since that time her hearing "comes and goes" and will often "fade away in the middle of a conversation." Behavioral deterioration was acknowledged by the parents.

On examination, there were no positive physical findings and audiometry demonstrated no response in the right ear. Pure tone levels of 80 to 90 dB with a 50 dB Speech Reception Threshold (SRT) and 96 per cent discrimination were identified in the left ear. Stenger tests were positive and communicative skills were inconsistent with thresholds.

Concerned for her daughter's hearing problems and in the absence of a specific diagnosis, the mother was distraught and was contemplating litigation against the physician and nurse who prescribed and administered the meperidol, respectively.

Under diazepam sedation, BERA confirmed normal thresholds bilaterally. This finding obviated further time-consuming and expensive evaluation, while clearly establishing future therapeutic direction. She is at this time progressing well under psychiatric management.

Attention is being directed toward increasing the amount of information generated by BERA in hard-to-test situations. Currently available BERA equipment and techniques yield accurate estimates of frequency-specidic threshold sensitivity.[1,7] Although BERA is still not able to supply information equal in scope to that generated by speech audiometry, prediction of pure tone audiogram shape using BERA would greatly expand the objective capabilities of this format. Its contribution to the clinical evaluation of auditory ability of infants and other difficult or inconsistent test subjects would also be enhanced. Implied is the importance of the pure tone audiogram to diagnosis and specifically to rehabilitation through amplification.

Don and colleagues,[30] acknowledging the problems in using BERA to predict or reconstruct audiogram shape, have recently proposed using a high-pass masking technique to analyze the function of the various frequency regions within the cochlea. Using a click stimulus, they clearly demonstrated the inadequacies of evaluating the apical regions of the cochlea responsible for low-tone contributions to auditory function. Filtered clicks,[31] tone pips, and tone bursts[32-34] similarly have been shown to exhibit serious shortcomings in estimating audiogram reconstruction.

By presenting clicks in high-pass masking noise and by varying the high-pass cut-off, the frequency-specific activity from the unmasked portion of the cochlear partition can be analyzed. Using all of the advantages of the click stimulus, specifically the synchrony it elicits and a moderately complicated protocol, frequency-specific information can be clearly generated.[30] Don and colleagues declared "a reasonably accurate reconstruction of the pure tone audiogram" as a potentially practical consideration. The information generated would be of monumental importance in the auditory rehabilitation of infants, of the mentally handicapped, or of any others in whom frequency-specific information is not otherwise available.

Reconstruction of audiogram shape using BERA would nicely compliment the auditory information compiled by a plot of latency-intensity functions. Hecox and Galambos[3] and Galambos and Hecox[35], as well as Brackmann[7] have demonstrated the capability of latency-intensity functions in the differentiation of sensory (neural) from conductive losses. These two contributions of BERA to the auditory evaluation significantly expand the restricted capability of "threshold determination" and what it means to auditory rehabilitation.

BERA, then, presents itself as an objective and accurate determination of auditory thresholds in hard-to-test situations commonly represented as behavioral failures. Screening of neonatal and infant high-risk groups, evaluation of young children, the mentally and physically handicapped, and those functional hearing-loss patients all represent important clinical applications. In any situation in which the generation of standard auditory data is inconsistent or deliberately complicated by patient inability or unwillingness to cooperate, behavioral formats can be confidently reinforced by BERA. Nonetheless, BERA is not a "hearing test" in that cortical integrative function is not evaluated. Its reliability and accuracy, however, clearly make it a practical inclusion into the clinical battery of auditory threshold tests.

Site of Lesion

A number of investigators have reported the diagnostic value of BERA in localizing lesions causing neurotological disorders.[1,10-12] BERA is particularly useful as a diagnostic adjunct in the evaluation of neurotological disease affecting the peripheral end-organ and its central projections up to and including the auditory brain stem pathways. Its proven reliability and retest accuracy confirms BERA's place in the neurotologic test battery.

As noted previously, distinguishing cochlear versus retrocochlear pathology is the crucial concern of site-of-lesion determination. BERA allows us to further subdivide the retrocochlear apparatus to consider lesions of the eighth nerve and brain stem. In the differential diagnosis of vertigo and hearing loss, the finer determination of site of lesion, in view of the commonness of these symptoms, is quite appealing.

The differential diagnosis of vertigo is not concise. Specific diagnosis is never simple. Meniere's disease must be differentiated from other etiologies, specifically acoustic tumor, other eighth nerve lesions, and brain stem disease. When a clinical diagnosis of Meniere's disease cannot be established or retrocochlear disease is not suspected, primary brain stem pathology, either neoplasia or demyelination, must be differentiated from other forms of non-Meniere's vertigo such as vestibular neuronitis, labyrinthine ischemia, positional vertigo, or functional disturbances. This is a common clinical dilemma often encountered in the presentation of the unsteady young female. BERA has demonstrated itself as a major contributor in the diagnostic confrontation of the serious afflictions, acoustic tumor and multiple sclerosis.

In assessing unilateral sensorineural hearing loss, the clinician must again entertain the diagnosis of acoustic tumor. Shia and Sheehy,[36] in their series of 1200 cases of unilateral sudden hearing loss, reported an incidence of acousic tumor in 0.8 percent. in such cases, BERA compliments behavioral indices of cochlear versus retrocochlear site of lesion. Furthermore, BERA subdivides the rectrocochlear apparatus into both neural and central brain stem projections. This capability has important implications when amplification is considered as therapy.

The accuracy of BERA in determining the presence of retrocochlear eighth nerve pathology in the form of acoustic tumor exceeded 95 per cent in the series reported by Glasscock and colleagues[11] and Selters and Brackmann.[9] Compression, stretching, or imposed ischemia of the auditory nerve as a result of the mass effects of these tumors alters neural transmission. It is this alteration in eighth nerve neurophysiology that is detected by BERA. Some tests in the site-of-lesion test battery accomplish this detection better than others, but BERA emerges superior in its reliability and sensitivity (see Chapter 3). In the absence of these mass effects, early diagnosis is virtually impossible and is usually made serendipitously.

A tumor mass effect is suspected when the generated responses of BERA demonstrate dysynchrony and wave V abnormalities. Dysynchrony is reflected principally in amplitude changes as well as in latency analysis of wave V and its relationship to preceding wave forms. Prolonged wave V latency represents the most sensitive detector of eighth nerve dysfunction. Brackmann and Selters achieve an improvement in test sensitivity by comparing wave V latencies in both ears (IT_5).[9] IT_5 for most patients is 0 msec, and in no case was there more than a 0.2-msec discrepancy.

However, as further experience was accrued, these authors revised their thinking regarding their original suggestion that IT_5 may be a reliable indicator of tumor size.[37] Correlation of IT_5 with tumor size has not been as consistent as originally expected. Displacement of the brain stem by large lesions often creates abnormalities in brain stem function, particularly when analyzed in the contralateral auditory system, a possibility even when the involved ear shows no auditory responsiveness. Selters reports such "off side" abnormalities in 77 per cent of 55 tumors 3 cm or larger.[37] He adds AP preservation (wave) in the absence of all other wave forms as a possible clue to the presence of a large cerebellopontine angle tumor as detected by BERA in all of 18 such cases in which this data pattern was acknowledged. Although not definitively diagnostic, this information may often be clinically useful to the otoneurosurgeon.

BERA is the most sensitive and accurate diagnostic test for acoustic tumor. False-negative rates are low and false-positive information is uniformly less than 10 percent.[9,11] In addition, no other test protocol generates more primary or objective information relative to the status of the brain stem.

The dissection of the concept of "retrocochlear" into eighth nerve and brain stem considerations proposes BERA as effective in the diagnosis of primary brain stem disorders, insofar as they affect brain stem auditory function. Starr[12] and Nodar[38] reported the accuracy of BERA not only in the detection of brain stem lesions but also in the precise localization of the anatomical site of specific lesions within the brain stem. Abnormalities of individual wave forms can be clinically interpreted as representing pathology at the site of its anatomical correlate, so that focal lesions can be precisely localized. The diffuse demyelinization of multiple sclerosis is objectively confirmed by extensive, variable wave form dysynchrony, whereas discrete lesions generate more specific patterns. For instance, a midbrain glioma might ablate waves IV and V selectively, whereas wave I might be the only wave form in evidence in a brain stem diffusely involved by multiple sclerosis.[11,39]

When considering retrocochlear auditory dysfunction, interpretation of data can be problematical. In addition to acoustic tumor, other etiologies of eighth nerve dysfunction include metabolic effects, selective fiber depopulation, degeneration, ischemia, or any other influence that might alter neural transmission. BERA is able to accurately and sensitively define, as well as localize, auditory dysfunction to the retrocochlear apparatus. It cannot, however, relate a histopathological diagnosis. The point to be made is that all that is "retrocochlear" in BERA testing, need not represent acoustic tumor in all cases. Indeed, the highest incidence of false diagnosis is generated within the context of evaluating the possibility of acoustic tumor in the presence of sensorineural insensitivity. In such circumstances, we have described a false-positive incidence of 9 per cent,[11] while Selters[37] has suggested, combining his false-positive and tumor incidence figures, an expectation of ten false-positive cases for every tumor diagnosis made when dealing with sudden sensorineural, unilateral loss. Since no acoustic tumor could be identified in these cases, test data were indeed falsely positive. It might be more appropriate, however, in light of BERA's accuracy and sensitivity, to refer to this data as "unsubstantiated" positive as opposed to "falsely" positive. Pathology obviously exists. It is, however, not the result of acoustic tumor.

Similarly, when brain stem auditory pathways are involved by neurotologic disease, wave V may be abnormally latent or totally absent with any number of variations existing in preceding wave forms. Does this data represent acoustic tumor, brain stem disease, or a primary deficit in neural transmission? BERA cannot be counted upon, singly, to accurately answer this question. BERA simply defines the existence of a problem, confirms the magnitude of its effect on auditory function, and localizes it within the auditory pathway. The term "simply" here, admittedly, represents a monumental understatement, for when interpreted within the enlightened context of the remainder of the neurotological evaluation a significant contribution has been made. For instance, absence of wave V, dilation of an internal auditory meatus, reduction of vestibular response, and a positive CAT scan clearly define the problem as an eighth nerve lesion. Conversely, the absence of wave V, normal behavioral audiometric data, normal internal auditory canals, "central" balance testing values and negative posterior fossa myelography strongly suggests primary brain stem disease. With the addition of BERA to the test battery, the clinician's high index of suspicion is confirmed far earlier and more accurately than ever before.

These problems must be specifically kept in mind when the unilateral, sensorineural losses of Meniere's disease are subjected to diagnostic scrutiny. These losses, however, are most generally low tone in character. It is decrements in hearing confined to the higher frequencies that present BERA with its highest hurdles. Apparently cochlear lesions have little effect on latency function or central conduction time in this pathway once the phenomenon of cochlear delay has been managed by achieving adequate stimulus parameters.[11] This fact is used in defining cochlear sites of lesion and differentiating them from latency extending retrocochlear problems. When the etiology of sensorineural hearing loss is not confirmed by standard audiometrics or when the diagnosis is not known at the onset,

BERA remains accurate in determining the site of lesion, as well as confirming the degree of loss.

The necessity of incorporating BERA into an organized protocol composed of a battery of tests must be re-emphasized. The presented limitations as well as the complicated sophistication of BERA, which can subject its data to misinterpretation in the hands of the inexperienced, make it essential to retain standard indicators for mutual reinforcement.

Case 5

D.A., a 17-year-old white male, presented with no neurotologic complaint, but his family history demonstrated evidence of von Recklinghausen's disease. He was referred for screening. His mother had bilateral eighth nerve neurolemmomas and an aunt recently underwent surgery for an accoustic tumor. The neurotologic work-up included pure tone and speech audiometry, petrous pyramid x-rays, electronystagmography (ENG), impedance audiometry with reflex testing and CAT scan. No abnormalities were detected. BERA test data revealed wave V to be absent on the left and delayed on the right (Fig. 4–2). With BERA representing the only positive test data, posterior fossa myelography was obtained. Bilateral acoustic tumors were identified. Middle fossa removal of one tumor failed to preserve hearing, whereas a similar approach to the contralateral lesion yielded excellent hearing results.

Comment: Preservation of hearing is a monumental achievement in these unfortunate patients who are often faced with the significant additional disability of diffuse neurofibromatosis within the neuraxis. This goal can be realized only through early diagnosis. BERA appears to afford, by virtue of its discrete sensitivity, the opportunity to effect early diagnosis not only in von

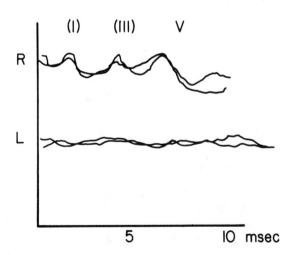

(I)   (III)   V

R

L

5   IO msec

Figure 4-2. BERA, case 5, D.A. See text for description. Absolute wave V latency on the right was 6.32 msec, clearly abnormal.

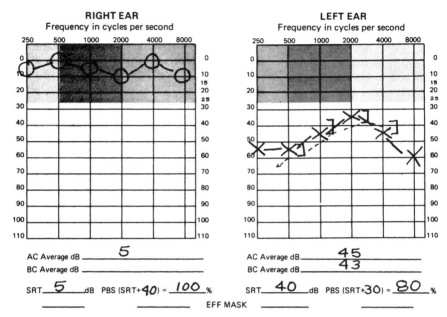

Figure 4–3. Audiogram, case 6, M.O. See text for description. Although typical of Meniere's disease, acoustical tumor must be ruled out.

Recklinghausen's disease, a rare entity, but also in the more common non-syndromic acoustic neuromata. Smaller lesions define lower morbidity and mortality associated with their management. The role of BERA as a screening device in these situations is proposed. Both of this patient's siblings had normal BERAs and similarly had no lesions on pantopaque myelography.

Case 6

M.O., a 39-year-old female, gave a 6-month history of aural fullness, fluctuant hearing, and recently, incapacitating, true, episodic vertigo associated with roaring tinnitus. All aural symptoms were left-sided.

Neurotologic examination was unremarkable. Pure-tone audiometry described a flat, sensorineural left loss of approximately 40 dB with 80 per cent discrimination (Fig. 4–3). Internal auditory canal x-rays, reflex decay, modified SISI and CAT scan were all unremarkable. ENG defined a minimally reduced left vestibular response. BERA confirmed the degree of loss and was otherwise normal. Steep latency-intensity function consistent with cochlear pathology was identified.

A diagnosis of left Meniere's disease was made and she now is being successfully managed medically.

Comment: The appropriate diagnosis was made clinically, but diagnostic exclusion of the possibility of accoustic tumor was essential. The established reliability of BERA associated with unquestioned normality of standard site-of-lesion tests in addition to no pathology on contrasted and unenhanced CAT scan allowed us to confidently exclude the diagnosis of cerebellopontine angle lesion noninvasively, that is, without the need for the hospitalization, expense, and potential morbidity of posterior fossa myelography.

Case 7

M.K., a 28-year-old bricklayer, had been unable to work for 2 weeks as a result of profound unsteadiness. He did not describe true, whirling vertigo but rather a constant disequilibrium. Hearing was diminished but subjectively was stable and of no significant social concern. He volunteered no other associated neurologic symptoms.

An ataxic gait and positive Romberg test were noted on examination. Puretone audiometry defined bilateral, flat sensorineural hearing losses of equal magnitude of approximately 35 dB (Fig. 4–4). Speech testing showed 90 per cent discrimination scores. ENG elaborated nonlocalizing findings that suggested central pathology. On BERA, wave I was identified bilaterally. Total dysynchrony of all subsequent characters was noted, no wave pattern being identifiable (Fig. 4–5). A diagnosis of multiple sclerosis was suggested, although it was impossible to confirm at that time, clinically.

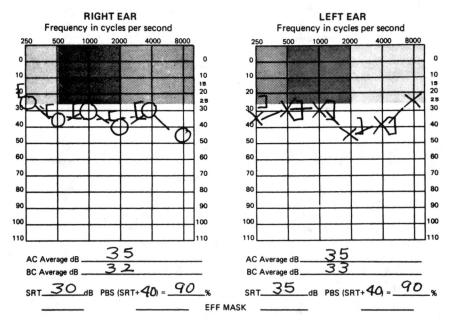

Figure 4–4. Audiogram, case 7, M.K. See text for description.

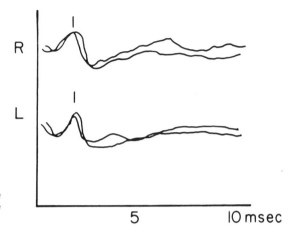

Figure 4-5. BERA, case 7, M.K. See text for description. A typical pattern representing the brain stem dysfunction of multiple sclerosis.

5   IO msec

Comment: The sensitivity of this indicator of brain stem dysfunction is established in this case. In the ensuing 2 weeks this patient went on to exhibit slurring of his speech, internuclear ophthalmoplegia and progressive neurological decompensation. Clinical confirmation of this dreaded diagnosis was then possible. BERA represents one of only few objective, totally noninvasive evaluations of brain stem integrity. Other currently available tests include visual evoked response and dark field adaptation studies.

In summary, BERA is very useful as a determinator of site of lesion in the neurotological context. Its profound sensitivity, objectivity, and noninvasive characteristics should promote its aggressive application.

SPECIAL CIRCUMSTANCES

In addition to confirmation of thresholds and standard site-of-lesion testing, the applicability of BERA in the clinical field has expanded as equipment and techniques have been improved. The following represent variations in the application of concepts of threshold testing and site-of-lesion determination to clinical situations more rarely encountered.

Berlin and colleagues[40] and Jerger[41] have applied the concepts of electric response audiometry to the resolution of masking dilemmas proposed often by those presenting bilateral conductive losses (Fig. 4-6). Clinically, these patients present certain problems, particularly if surgery is contemplated.[40] Is one ear anacoustic and the audiogram spurious? Is either loss purely sensorineural with air curve and bone curve equal? Impedance audiometry, tuning forks, and the SAL test might all potentially resolve this problem, but often poor patient cooperation or an inability to comprehend test procedures impose serious limitations on these formats.

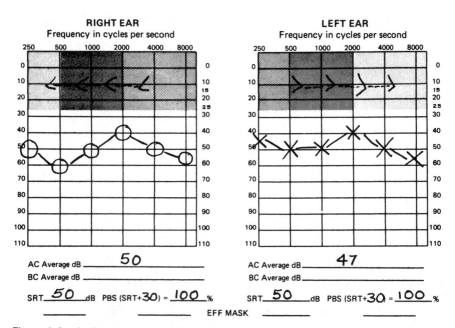

Figure 4-6. Audiogram, case 8, N.S. See text for details. Represented is the classic masking dilemma of bilateral conductive losses.

An objective indicator that bypasses the patient's subjective input, the problems of masking, and complicating interaural factors would reliably establish separately each ear's cochlear reserve.

As a result of the difficulties associated with the efficiency of air-conducted stimuli in these situations, the test apparatus must be modified so that a bone-conducted stimulus could be presented.[40] Cochlear function can then be directly evaluated, completely bypassing the conductive apparatus and the need for masking.

Masking dilemmas are not uncommon. Bilateral otosclerosis with conductive losses, extensive bilateral tympanosclerosis, congenital conductive losses, and bilateral cholesteatomata all pose problems, particularly in a preoperative circumstance when avoidance of an only-hearing or a better-hearing ear whenever possible is preferable. Bone-conducted BERA presents a protocol variation of classic site-of-lesion testing whose applicability and clinical usefulness cannot be understated.

Case 8

N.S. is a 58-year-old white female with bilateral otosclerosis. Her audiogram is shown in Figure 4-6. Weber was midline but inconsistent. Impedance audiometry yielded absent reflexes bilaterally. She was unable to subjectively isolate a "better ear." Surgery was suggested and desired by the patient.

Bone-conducted BERA demonstrated adequate and essentially equal cochlear reserve bilaterally so that either ear represented a surgical candidate. Right stapedectomy was successfully accomplished.
Comment: Again BERA served to effectively support a behavioral failure. If an audiogram had been spurious and an only-hearing ear had been operated on, particularly in stapes surgery, an otological disaster might have occurred. Similarly, if an anacoustic ear had been operated on, an unnecessary procedure would have exposed the patient unjustifiably to the well-known morbid risks of stapedectomy.

The use of BERA in the field of neurology has been expanded to include a role in the determination of brain death. The application of electric response audiometry, however, in this context is not new. Cortical responses and EEG data were measured in 1973 by Trojaborg and Jorgenson[42] in an attempt to diagnose brain death. Inconsistent and generally unreliable data were obtained. Starr, however, has suggested[43] BERA be included in the criteria of evaluation of brain death.

In conjunction with standard clinical criteria of brain death, Starr identified in 27 patients an absent brain stem response, wave I being the only wave character inconsistently preserved.[43] In addition, he was able to follow the progressive deterioration of brain stem function in four patients who sustained acute anoxic insults. Serial brain stem audiograms demonstrated first a normal pattern followed by dissolution of the wave IV–wave V complex only to subsequently note the loss of waves II and III, and an inconsistently demonstrated abnormality in wave I. Starr, nonetheless, correctly stressed the need for BERA to be evaluated within the context of the clinical evaluation of the comatose patient. BERA is only a reflection of a single sensory function that indirectly reflects the overall integrity of the brain stem. The deaf patient, the patient with primary pre-existing brain stem disease, and the complexity of the test confine this objective test to an adjunctive role, complimenting the patient's clinical evaluation, laboratory tests, and EEG. Auditory brain stem responses do, however, supply an objective measure of the functional status of the brain stem and in the circumstance surrounding a definition of brain death, provide data often helpful to the physician who is faced with the unenviable task of attempting to resolve this question.

Again as equipment and experience have matured, certain technical refinements to BERA have been suggested. In addition to the traditional analysis of wave V latency in the site-of-lesion scheme of BERA, determination of central conduction time, that is, the wave III to wave V or the wave I to wave V interval, has come to be respected as a very valuable and accurate indicator of retrocochlear pathology. Coats and Martin,[44] using the concepts of inappropriate AP preservation, have proposed an interesting technical modification.

In the far-field technique of BERA, wave I is often poorly defined, making analysis of central conduction times quite difficult, if not completely impossible. Coats and Martin[44] have, therefore, suggested routine clinical use of simultaneous recording of AP and BERA responses. In this context, a dual channel recording system recording data from both the auditory meatus (or promontory) and the vertex is necessary. The simultaneous recording of eighth nerve action potentials and brain stem auditory electric responses, therefore, represents a technical refinement that at this time appears useful in those circumstances in which analysis of central conduction time is crucial, but in which vertex far-field techniques fail to generate the appropriate data as a result of audiogram shape or other forms of auditory pathology.

By no means is the science of electric responses audiometry clinically static. Experience obtained within the last 5 to 10 years, both with the neurophysiology and the technical aspects of BERA, foreshadow the upcoming decade as one in which a clinical explosion of information in this regard can be expected.

REFERENCES

1. Davis, H.: Principles of electric response audiometry. Ann Otol Rhinol Laryngol 85(Suppl 79):1-96, 1976.
2. Jewett, D. L., Romano, H. N., and Williston, J. S.: Human auditory evoked responses: possible brainstem components detected on the scalp. Science 167:1517-1518, 1970.
3. Hecox, K., and Galambos, R.: Brainstem auditory evoked responses in human infants and adults. Arch Otolaryngol 99:30-33, 1974.
4. Starr, A., and Hamilton, A. E.: Correlation between confirmed sites of neurological lesions and abnormalities of far field auditory brainstem responses. Electroencephalog Clin Neurophysiol 41:595-608, 1976.
5. Stockard, J. T., and Rossiter, V. S.: Clinical and pathologic correlates of brainstem auditory response. Neurology 27:316-325, 1977.
6. Buchwald, J., and Huany, C. M.: Far field acoustic response: origins in the CAT. Science 189:382-384, 1975.
7. Brackmann, D. E.: Electric response audiometry in a clinical practice. Laryngoscope 87(Suppl 5):1-33, 1977.
8. Picton, T. W., Woods, D. L., Baribeau-Braun, B. A., and Healey, T. M. G.: Evoked potential audiometry. J. Otolaryngol 6:90-118, 1977.
9. Selters, W. A., and Brackmann, D. E.: Acoustic tumor detection with brainstem electric response audiometry. Arch Otolaryngol 103:181-187, 1977.
10. Clemis, J. D., and McGree, T.: Brainstem electric response audiometry in the differential diagnosis of acoustic tumors. Laryngoscope 89:31-42. 1979.
11. Glasscock, M. E., Jackson, C. G., Josey, A. F., Dickens, J. R. E., and Wiet, R. J.: Brainstem evoked response audiometry in clinical practice. Laryngoscope 89:1021-1034, 1979.

12. Starr, A., and Achor,L. J.: Auditory brainstem responses in neurologic disease. Arch Neurol 32:761–768, 1975.
13. Berlin, C. J., and Dobie, R. A.: Electrophysiological measures of auditory function via electrocochleograph and brainstem evoked response. Rintelmann, W. F. (ed.): *Hearing Assessment.* Baltimore, University Park Press, 1979.
14. Jerger, J., Mouldin, L., and Anthony, I.: Brainstem evoked response. audiometry. Audiol Hear Educ. 4:17–24, 1978.
15. Hecox, K., and Galambos, R.: Brainstem auditory evoked responses in human infants and adults. Arch Otolaryngol 99:30–33, 1974.
16. Witten, R., and Wade, C. T.: Computed tomography in acoustic tumor diagnosis. *Acoustic Tumors Volume I: Diagnosis,* pp. 253–277. Baltimore, University Park Press, 1979.
17. Davis, H., Hirsh, S. K., Shelnutt, J., Bowers, C.: Further validation of evoked response audiometry (ERA). J Speech Hear Res 10:717–732, 1967.
18. McCandless, G. A., and Best, L.: Evoked responses using puretone stimuli. J Speech Hear Res 9:266–272, 1966.
19. Rapin, I., Shimmel, H., Tourk, C. M., et. al.: Evoked responses to clicks and tones of varying intensity in waking adults. Electorencephalogr Clin Neurophysiol 21L335–344, 1966.
20. Skinner, P., and Glattke, T. J.: Electrophysiologic response audiometry: state of the art. J Speech Hear Dis 62:179–198, 1977.
21. Lentz, W. E., and McCandless, G. A.: Averaged electroencephalographic audiometry in infants. J Speech Hear Dis 36:19–28, 1971.
22. Schulman-Galambos, C., and Galambos, R.: Brainstem evoked response audiometry in newborn hearing screening. Arch Otolaryngol 105:86–90, 1979.
23. Cohen, J. J., Rapin, I., Lyttle, M., Shimmel, H.: Auditory evoked response (AER) consistency of detection in young sleeping children. Arch Otolaryngol 94:214–219, 1971.
24. Rapin, I., Schimmel, H., and Cohen, M. M.: Reliability in detecting the auditory evoked response (AER) for audiometry in sleeping subjects. Electroencephalogr Clin Neurophysiol 32:521–528, 1967.
25. Rise, D. E., Keating, L. W., Hedgecock, L. D., et. al.: A comparison of evoked response audiometry and routine clinical audiometry. Audiology 11:238–243, 1972.
26. Hume, A. L., and Cont, B. R.: Diagnosis of hearing loss in infancy by electric response audiometry. Arch Otolaryngol 103:416–418, 1977.
27. Mokotoff, M. A., Schulman-Galambos, C., and Galambos, R.: Brain stem auditory evoked responses in children. Arch Otolaryngol 103:38–43, 1977.
28. Hanley, C., and Tiffary, W. R.: Auditory malingering and psychogenic deafness. Arch Otolaryngol 60:197–201, 1954.
29. McCandless, G. A., and Lentz, W.: Evoked response (EEG) audiometry in non-organic hearing loss. Arch Otolaryngol 87:123–128, 1968.
30. Don, M., Eggermont, J. J., and Brackmann, D. E.: Reconstruction of the audiogram using brainstem responses and high pons noise masking. Ann Otol Rhinol Laryngol 88(Suppl 57): 1979.
31. Brama, I., and Sohmer, H.: Auditory nerve and brainstem responses to sound stimuli at various frequencies. Audiology 16:402–408, 1977.
32. Stillman, R. D., Monsshegian, G., and Rupert, A. L.: Early tone evoked responses in normal and hearing impaired subjects. Audiology 15:10–22, 1976.
33. Mitchell, C., and Clemis, J. D. Audiograms derived from brainstem response. Laryngoscope 87:2016–2022, 1977.
34. Davis, H., and Hirsh, S. K.: The audiometric utility of brain stem responses to low frequency sounds. Audiology 15:181–195, 1976.
35. Galambos, R., and Hecox, K.: Clinical applications of the human brainstem evoked potential to auditory stimuli. *In* Desmedt, J. E. (ed): *Progress in Clinical Neurophysiology, Vol. 2. Auditory Evoked Potentials in Man: Psychopneumocology Correlates of Evoked Potentials.* Basel, S. Karger, 1977.

36. Shia, F., and Sheehy, J.: Sudden sensorineural hearing impairment: a report of 1220 cases. Laryngoscope 86:389-398, 1976.
37. Selters, W. A., and Brackmann, D. E.: Brainstem electric response audiometry in acoustic tumor detection. *In* House, W. F. and Luetje, C. M. (eds): *Acoustic Tumors Volume I: Diagnosis,* pp. 225-235, Baltimore, University Park Press, 1979.
38. Nodár, R. H., Hahn, J., and Levine, H. L.: Brainstem auditory evoked potentials in determining site of lesion of brainstem gliomas in children. Laryngoscope 90:258-265, 1980.
39. Robinson, K., and Rudge, P.: Abnormalities of the auditory evoked potentials in patients with multiple sclerosis. Brain 100:19-40, 1977.
40. Berlin, C. I., Cullen, J. K.: Clinical experience with electrocochleography: special applications in bone conduction. *In* Shea, J. J. and Gambaugh, G. E. (eds): *Proceedings of the Shambaugh Fifth International Workshop on Middle Ear Microsurgery and Fluctuant Hearing Loss,* pp. 68-74. Alabama, Strode Publishers, Inc., 1977.
41. Jerger, J., Mouldin, L., and Anthony, I.: Brainstem evoked response audiometry. Audiol Hear Educ. 4:17-24, 1978.
42. Trojaborg, W., and Jorgenson, E. O.: Evoked cortical potentials in patients with isoelectric EEGs. Electroencephalogr Clin Neurophysiol 35:301-309, 1973.
43. Starr, A.: Auditory brainstem responses in brain death. Brain 99:543-554, 1976.
44. Coats, A. C., and Martin, J. L. Human auditory nerve action potentials and brainstem evoked responses. Arch Otolaryngol 103:605-622, 1977.

Chapter Five

CLINICAL RESULTS OF BERA

INTRODUCTION

Brain stem electric response audiometry (BERA) is a sensitive electrophysiological measure of the integrity of the auditory system from end-organ through the brain stem. Clinically, the test has been firmly established to be useful in several situations (see Chapter 4), identifying both sensitively and accurately the effects of neurotologic disease on the neurophysiology of this system. Selters and Brackman[1] and Glasscock and colleagues[2] have stressed applicability to site-of-lesion testing, the emphasis being neurotologic. Starr[3,4] and Stockard and Rossiter[5] have evaluated site of lesion from within the field of neurology. Others, notably Hecox and Galambos,[6] Jerger,[7] and Berlin,[8] have established its reliability, objectivity, and limitations in the assessment of peripheral threshold sensitivity. It was in this regard that BERA was originally incorporated into the established testing protocol designed to evaluate neurotologic disease in our practice. Over the subsequent 2 years well over 500 patients had their neurotologic complaints evaluated by our conventional battery of tests with the addition of BERA. This chapter presents the results of this clinical experience.

METHOD

Although Chapter 3 presented a significantly more detailed demonstration of those principles and methods germane to the generation and interpretation of data by BERA, a more basic technical statement is indicated here. A summary, therefore, of our method previously described[2] is included.

The vast majority of patients included in this analysis were tested in a clinical setting, which generally afforded them a quiet, comfortable environment (Fig. 5-1). The test was administered by an audiologist without physician supervision and was performed in an unshielded room, the patient usually in a reclining position. The administration of adjunctive seda-

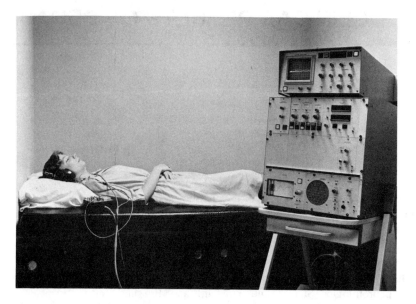

Figure 5-1. Patient testing should be in a quiet, comfortable setting.

tion or any medication, other than that which was being taken for unrelated medical problems or the pathophysiological process under investigation, was generally not necessary. Six adults, however, required diazepam to reduce sonomotor contaminants in the recording at some time prior to test completion. General anesthesia was used only to effect threshold testing in those infants not otherwise controllable in the test circumstance, an infrequent occurrence. Most adult patients simply fell asleep, and infants were generally tested immediately after feeding.

Gold scalp electrodes were applied, defining the vertex as the active and the ipsilateral mastoid as the inactive or reference site. The contralateral mastoid served as ground. Interelectrode resistances were balanced, and electrode resistance was maintained at under 5000 ohms. Modification of electrode procedures became necessary to accomodate artifacts generated from monitoring equipment, steel cranial prostheses, coronary pacemakers, and so forth.

Clinical test equipment included the Life Tech 8101 BERA stimulus generator and signal energizer. Acoustic transients to clicks of 0.1-millisecond (msec) duration were presented through shielded TDH 39 earphones at intensities no lower than 75 decibel hearing level (dB HL) relative to a jury of ten normal-hearing young adults. In order to accommodate variations in end-organ sensitivity, stimulus parameters were occasionally altered. Click presentation or repetition rate was maintained at eight per second, averaging 1024 stimulus-response cycles per average. A dwell time, or gate, of 10 msec was employed.

In addition to wave V latency, analysis of central conduction times became possible with improved definition of waves I, III, and occasionally VI. Amplitude changes of binaural summation were qualitatively evaluated. Wave V latency was compared to a mean normal of 5.4 msec (range 5.1 to 5.9 msec) and was suspected to be abnormal if it exceeded 6.0 msec only when stimulus characteristics achieved peak latency of wave V. This limit was extended upward to 6.2 msec for normal-hearing subjects older than age 55 years. When available, wave I latency was used to analyze central conduction time (waves I to V), the more sensitive indicator of retrocochlear pathology. In this population, normal central conduction time ranged from 3.8 to 4.2 msec with a mean of 4.0 msec. A central conduction time in excess of 4.4 msec was identified as a significant abnormality. Interaural differences were reviewed according to the criteria established by Selters and Brackmann.[7] In some cases, latency-intensity functions were plotted to provide further differentiation of site of lesion in the periphery as described by Jerger.[9] Retest latency reliability served to establish response validity. Response amplitude was qualitatively acknowledged only for marked interaural discrepancies.

CLINICAL MATERIAL

In the 2-year period from January 1977 to December 1978 we evaluated more than 500 patients, with BERA contributing clinical information. This group represents the first 500 cases on whom sufficient clinical data and follow-up exists to substantiate their clinical diagnoses. Histopathology is available in some cases. Excluded are those patients tested in consultation only or those who were lost to follow-up.

The character of the neurotologic practice of The Otology Group predefined site-of-lesion testing as the most common situation of applicability for BERA. However, BERA was requested in evaluating basically four clinical circumstances: (1) patients in whome initial audiologic data suggested a need for further site-of-lesion testing, (2) patients in whom standard behavioral formats failed as a result of failure or inability to cooperate or comprehend basic testing procedures, (3) malingerers or patients whose test data were inconsistent, and (4) patients in whom primary neurologic brain stem disease was suspected. For most of these cases additional audiologic, radiologic, and vestibulographic data was available for comparison with that generated by BERA.

Based on clinical diagnosis and objective substantiation, the population under study was grouped into the following categories: (1) lesions of the internal auditory canal or cerebellopontine angle, (2) Meniere's disease, (3) non-Meniere's vertigo, (4) sensorineural hearing loss, (5) primary brain stem disorders, (6) confirmation of threshold, and (7) miscellaneous (facial paralysis, otalgia, tinnitus, and so forth).

RESULTS

Group 1: Lesions of the Internal Auditory Canal or Cerebellopontine Angle

This first group was composed of 60 surgically confirmed lesions exhibited by 59 patients whose clinical situation was amenable to BERA testing. One patient had von Recklinghausen's disease and presented bilateral acoustic neurinomata. Within this time frame an additional nine lesions were diagnosed, all acoustic tumors, none of which was a candidate for BERA analysis. Eight of these nine patients demonstrated no audiological response below 500 Hz, the ninth patient demonstrated no detectable preoperative hearing. All nine patients were tested for "off side" abnormalities.

The population of this group included 34 males and 25 females ranging in age from 16 to 63 years (mean 42.1 years). Histologically, 57 acoustic neurinomata were identified. The remaining three unusual lesions were defined as (1) a cholesteatoma, (2) a papilloma of the choroid plexus, and (3) an angioblastic meningioma. Of the 57 acoustic tumors, 14 were small lesions (up to 1.5 cm), 34 were tumors of medium size (1.5 to 4.0 cm) and 9 lesions were 4 cm or larger.

All patients in this group were studied to varying degrees using those diagnostic tests that compose our neurotologic battery designed to evaluate and define the nature of clinically suspected retrocochlear pathol-

TABLE 5–1.

PTA	N	PB Range	Mean
0–25	13	56–100	88.6
26–35	5	14–100	70.0
36–45	14	12–96	56.7
46–55	12	0–90	49.9
56–65	5	0–82	42.8
66–75	8	0–48	28.4
76–	3	0–22	14.0

TABLE 5–2.

	SISI		TDT		IRD		BERA	
	N	%	N	%	N	%	N	%
Retrocochlear pathology								
suggested	39	66.1	43	72.9	49	81.6	59	98.3
Nonretrocochlear	20	33.9	16	27.1	11	19.4	1	1.7

SISI - Short Increment Sensitivity Index   IRD - Impedance Reflex Decay   TDT - Tone Decay Testing
BERA - Brain Stem Electric Response Audiometry

ogy. This diagnostic protocol includes (1) a complete neurotologic historical review and physical examination, (2) an audiologic evaluation and, when indicated, BERA, (3) plain x-rays of the internal auditory canal and again, when appropriate unenhanced and contrasted computed axial tomography (CAT) scanning of the head, and (4) electronystagmography (ENG). Posterior fossa myelography (PFM) was occasionally necessary to confirm small turmor diagnosis.

Audiologic data included pure tone and speech results, impedance audiometry, modified Short Increment Sensitivity Index (SISI), Olsen modification of the Carhart tone decay test, and BERA. On pure tone testing, mean pure tone average ranged from 0 dB to 76 dB with a mean of 50 dB. Mean speech discrimination score was 55.6 percent, representing a wide range from 0 to 100 per cent. Table 5–1 summarizes these results relative to degree of loss. Comparative analysis of the efficacy of the other audiological tests, including BERA, in this circumstance is presented in Table 5–2.

All audiologic tests were found consistent with a diagnosis of retrocochlear pathology in only 29 cases or 48.3 percent of these surgically confirmed lesions. All tests were falsely negative (including BERA) in a single patient (1.7 percent). BERA results were surgically corroborated in all 60 of these lesions.

The definitive diagnosis of cerebellopontine angle lesion was roentgenographically established in all cases by either CAT scanning or posterior fossa myelography. Radiological data is summarized in Table 5–3. The bias of this group toward the smaller lesion is reflected in the unimpressive performance of CAT scanning in this population.

TABLE 5–3.

Study	Normal		Abnormal		N
PPX	10	(20.8%)	38	(79.2%)	48
CAT	24	(48.0%)	26	(52.0%)	50
PFM	0	(0%)	43	(100.0%)	43

ENG is a relatively nonlocalizing evaluation in the cochlear versus retrocochlear context and is, therefore, considered separately. ENG was available in 41 patients, being consistent with peripheral pathology in 78.9 percent, normal in 14.6 percent, and nonlocalizing or central in 7.4 percent.

Comment

It is readily apparent from an analysis of these data on surgically confirmed lesions of the internal auditory canal and cerebellopontine angle that BERA emerges as the most accurate audiometric test for acoustic tumor detection. Clearly warranted is its inclusion in the site-of-lesion protocol. The sensitivity of BERA, which is nearly as important as its accuracy, merits acknowledgment in consideration of the concept of early diagnosis.

Even in those small lesions in which hearing is normal and other special tests are unrevealing, BERA has been shown to demonstrate sufficient sensitivity to identify eighth nerve lesions with a high rate of success.[9] Table 5-4 represents a comparison of the sensitivity of the various special tests including BERA when considering these types of lesions.

Although the accuracy of the other special tests increases with the degree of loss, BERA compares favorably with the addition of accurately detecting the presence of acoustic tumor in 13 normal hearing instances. Falsely negative data was generated in only a single case. Referred for the evaluation of unilateral tinnitus, pure tone and speech audiometry as well as all special audiometric tests were unremarkable. CAT scan and ENG similarly contributed little to a diagnosis. A dilated internal auditory canal however was identified on plain films. Posterior fossa myelography subsequently demonstrated a 1.5 cm lesion, histologically an acoustic neu-

TABLE 5–4.

PTA	N	Mod SISI + %	Mod SISI False − %	TDT + %	TDT False − %	IRD + %	IRD False − %	BERA Delay %	BERA Abs %	BERA False − %
0–25	13	38.5	61.5	30.8	69.2	46.1	53.9	69.1	29.2	1.7
26–35	5	40.0	60.0	40.0	60.0	100.0	0.0	60.0	40.0	0.0
36–45	14	84.6	15.4	76.9	23.1	92.8	7.2	7.1	92.9	0.0
46–55	12	83.3	17.7	83.3	17.7	100.0	0.0	8.3	91.7	0.0
56–65	5	80.0	20.0	80.0	20.0	80.0	20.0	20.0	80.0	0.0
66–75	8	100.0	0.0	75.0	25.0	100.0	0.0	0.0	100.0	0.0
76–	3	100.0	0.0	100.0	0.0	100.0	0.0	0.0	100.0	0.0

TABLE 5–5.

Diagnosis:	Meniere's Disease	SNHL	Vertigo	Miscellaneous
N:	221	188	102	53
Test:				
SISI	6.6%	11.0%	DNT	DNT
TDT	8.4%	9.5%	DNT	DNT
IRD	8.7%	8.8%	1.8%	10.8%
BERA	4.1%	9.6%	2.0%	5.7%

SNHL - Sensorineural Hearing Loss

rinoma. The growth characteristics of this particular lesion obviously imposed little, if any, dysfunction in the auditory system capable of being detected by standard modern technology. The importance of the test battery is emphasized.

It is important to consider the concept of false-negative data as it relates to histopathology. Admittedly, the false-negative incidence reported in this series is quite low and inconsistent with that reported by Selters and Brackmann.[1] The diversity of the histopathology that composed his population must be acknowledged, and it is within this subgroup of "nonacoustic" cerebellopontine angle lesions that falsely negative information is most commonly generated. Our lack of experience with these more unusual pathological entities probably accounts for the data presented herein. Consideration of this point serves to further emphasize the necessity of maintaining a battery of tests that compliment and reinforce one another.

Retrospectively analyzing a group of patients exhibiting surgically confirmed lesions introduces a bias in selecting against these cases in which BERA was otherwise misleading, generating falsely positive information. False-positive findings occur for BERA as well as for other components of the diagnostic protocol designed to evaluate site of lesion. Table 5–5 summarized the results in this series.[2,9]

Clearly, the highest incidence of this falsely positive information occurs in the analysis of undifferentiated sensorineural hearing loss. It is, however, not unreasonable to assume that a given proportion of these losses represent neural or central auditory dysfunction and that the BERA data may well represent unsubstantiated rather than falsely positive retrocochlear localization. Nonetheless, the limits of our diagnostic technology and capabilities clearly impose this inaccuracy upon us and regardless of whether we call it unsubstantiated or false, the generated data still mislead us. Such an acknowledgment requires empirical definition. Overall, the incidence of false-positive information generated by BERA in all groups is approximately 5.3 percent. This figure agrees with 8 percent incidence reported by Selters and Brackmann.[1] The fact remains that this data for BERA compares quite favorably with that generated by other tests in the protocol.

The other limitations of electric response audiometry as applied to site-of-lesion testing and already discussed in the preceding chapter should be re-emphasized. BERA is severely limited in its application when severe or profound high tone sensorineural losses are encountered, a circumstance not uncommon when acoustic tumor is a diagnostic possibility. The inability of BERA to define type of pathology similarly represents a relative limitation. BERA is simply unable to define the pathological etiology of the abnormal physiology that it so sensitively and accurately is able to localize. Definition of demyelinating, degenerative, or neoplastic influence exceeds that which can reasonably be expected of BERA in site-of-lesion testing.

Keeping well in mind its limitations, BERA represents a monumental contribution to the effectiveness of the neurotologic test battery, Nonetheless, test limitations relegate BERA to an adjunctive role in this battery. The reliable performance of impedance audiometry and acoustic reflex decay suggests it be routinely applied. Similarly, tone decay and SISI tests ably reinforce BERA in these instances of high-frequency hearing losses. Radiologic substantiation of the diagnosis of acoustic tumor is essential, but equally important is the role of x-ray in supporting BERA in the identification of these "nonacoustic" lesions that may, or often may not, alter auditory physiology to a detectable degree. It must be remembered that posterior fossa myelography is still the most accurate detector of acoustic tumors. BERA, however, is firmly established as the most accurate noninvasive indicator of retrocochlear pathology, and its contribution to the test battery is obvious.

The roentgenographic data, particularly with regard to the success of CAT scanning in defining this type of pathology, deserves comment. Selection of this series to evaluate success of BERA biases the data by selecting better hearing cases, which generally implies lesions smaller in size. The resolving power of CAT scanning rarely exceeds definition of lesions smaller than 1.5 cm.[10] We would therefore suggest that the figure of 52 percent accuracy presented here is probably unjustifiably low. Witten and Wade for instance describe a false-negative incidence in their total series of 13 percent.[10] It was their expressed opinion that 90 percent of acoustic tumors larger than 1.5 cm are diagnosed by CAT scan. However, tumors smaller than 1.5 cm are accurately defined with this method only 50 percent of the time.

In summary, BERA appears to be the best test for the detection of acoustic tumors and other Cerebellopotine (CPA) lesions. Its reliability, sensitivity, and accuracy is established. Its role as a screening test is pro-posed. An inability to define the type of pathology and the concept of the untestable ear represent limitations for BERA, so standard diagnostic for-mats should not be supplanted. BERA presents itself as a powerful adjunct to the neurotologic diagnosis of retrocochlear pathology and has served in-valuably in the evaluation of subsequent groups of patients in which the diagnosis of acoustic tumor had to be excluded.

Group 2: Meniere's Disease

Included in this group are those patients to whom the clinical diag-nosis of Meniere's disease has been appended based on the criteria estab-lished by the American Academy of Otolaryngology.[11] Cochlear and ves-tibular hydrops, although rare, were included. One hundred seventy-six patients presented 221 pathological ears, and a slight female predominance was identified (100 females; 76 males). These patients ranged in age from 9 to 73 years with a mean of 45.5 years. The incidence of bilateral disease was 26 percent.

Audiologically, the average pure tone average was 38.3 dB (HTL), with a range of 3.3 to 91.5 dB HTL, whereas the average PB score was 79.7 percent ranging from 0 to 100 percent. Special tests results including BERA are shown in Table 5–6. Radiological data is also presented.

In this group, 208 ears were evaluated by ENG. Again, although nonlocalizing in regard to cochlear versus retrocochlear localization, 111 (52.8 percent) demonstrated peripheral pathology, and in 19 (9.1 percent) central pathology was suggested. No abnormality was identified in 58 (27.9 percent), and results were nonlocalizing in 20 instances (9.6 per-cent).

Comment

Meniere's disease is a common presenting disorder in which the dif-ferential diagnosis often includes possible retrocochlear pathology, more

TABLE 5–6.

	SISI	TDT	BERA	IRD	CAT	PPX	PFM
N:	91	107	221	173	165	186	67
Normal retrocochlear apparatus suggested	93.4%	91.6%	95.9%	91.3%	100%	91.4%	98.5%
Retrocochlear pathology suggested	6.6%	8.4%	4.1%	8.7%	0	7.5%	1.5%

CAT - Computed Axial Tomography   PPX - Petrous Pyramid X-rays   PFM - Posterior Fossa Myelogram commonly acoustic tumor but primary brain stem disorders as well. These considerations must be excluded from the clinical picture before a therapeutic protocol can be formulated to deal effectively with the peripheral process of Meniere's disease. Occasionally, such an exclusion process is quite difficult, but ostensibly, BERA has made many contributions toward the objective, noninvasive resolution of this problem. Here, also, the data represent BERA as the most accurate audiological indicator of site of lesion in this group.

Apparently cochlear lesions have little effect on latency functions and central conduction times in this pathway once the phenomenon of cochlear delay imposed by the hearing loss is managed.[2] More severe hearing losses, it seems, impose limitations on the efficiency of BERA in this context. In six patients, BERA data had to be reported as nonlocalizing as a result of test problems created by severe hearing losses (high frequency predominantly). By definition, this information must be reported as falsely positive. If, however, these six are excluded as "nonlocalizing," the false-positive incidence falls to only 1.4 percent as opposed to the 4.1 percent reported, which includes these patients. Three patients, nonetheless, suggested retrocochlear pathology in the presence of no more than a moderate loss. It appears then that a small percentage of Meniere's patients will present misleading data on BERA but that more severe hearing losses introduce significant problems relative to the generation of reliable data. In these few cases the severity of cochlear pathology most probably prohibits the synchrony of cochlear discharge so necessary to successful evaluation of the retrocochlear system.[2] Nonetheless, emphasis must be appropriately applied to the comparison of the data generated by BERA with that of other standard test. BERA emerges quite favorably superior to more conventional noninvasive formats.

BERA, as outlined in the preceding chapter, has contributed, in this context, to a streamlining of the evaluation of these patients with Meniere's disease toward a noninvasive emphasis. A cochlear site-of-lesion localization on BERA taken with a normal CAT scan as well as an unremarkable remainder of the neurotologic test battery confers a highly accurate exclusion of retrocochlear pathology. These data, then, justify the preclusion of posterior fossa myelography, an obviously invasive agent.

Group 3: Non-Meniere's Vertigo

This group was composed of those cases in which a clinical diagnosis of Meniere's disease could not be established, but in which vertigo was a prevalent problem. Included, for example, were vestibular neuronitis, labrinthine ischemia, benign positional vertigo, and so forth. One hundred

TABLE 5–7.

	BERA	IRD	CAT	PPX	PFM
N:	102	57	60	93	15
Normal retrocochlear apparatus suggested	98.0%	98.2%	100%	81.3%	100%
Retrocochlear pathology suggested	2.0%	1.8%	0	18.7%	0

two patients—52 females and 50 males—were so categorized. Their ages ranged from 13 to 73 years, with a mean of 44.9 years.

Audiologically, pure tone average was 15 dB HTL with an average speech discrimination score of 92.2 percent. The results of testing, including BERA, are summarized in Table 5-7.

ENG in 100 of these cases demonstrated a normal tracing in 26 percent, peripheral pathology in 30 percent, and results suggesting central or nonlocalizing pathology in 44 percent.

Comment

BERA was consistent, in all but two cases, with the remainder of the neurotologic evaluation. In this context BERA served as an important adjunct in the evaluation of retrocochlear pathology, specifically acoustic tumor or primary brain stem disease, so often questioned in this group of patients in whom peripheral vestibular pathology is not often as clearly evident as it might be in Meniere's disease.

In analyzing the two patients (2 percent) with unconfirmed abnormal data on BERA, both demonstrated abnormal responses at wave III or later. One patient carried a diagnosis of vertebrobasilar insufficiency and an unconfirmed diagnosis of brain stem infarction. The second subject exhibited on the right a normal wave V but on the left only wave I with a questionable wave III at 4.8 msec, a pattern suggestive of brain stem pathology. It might well be that these two "false positives" are actually truly "unsubstantiated positives" representing neurologically unconfirmed brain stem pathology diagnosable in no other way.

Group 4: Sensorineural Hearing Loss

One hundred twenty-one subjects and 188 pathologic ears composed this group of patients who presented a sensorineural hearing loss to which a

TABLE 5–8.

	SISI	TDT	BERA	IRD	CAT	PPX	PFM
N:	129	147	188	171	116	55	56
Normal retrocochlear apparatus suggested	89.0%	90.5%	90.4%	91.2%	100%	91.6%	100%
Retrocochlear pathology suggested	11.0%	9.5%	9.6%	8.8%	0	8.4%	0

diagnosis could be ascribed. They included congenital losses, those thought to be hereditary, and those losses that were ototoxic, leutic, noise-induced, or viral such as measles (Rubella) or mumps. Presbycusis was included. Sixty-nine females and 57 males averaged 43.6 years of age (range 7 to 69 years).

Pure tone averages ranged from 8.9 to 85.0 dB, with a mean of 38.4 dB and average speech scores of 78.3 percent. No patient exhibited auditory function that could not be tested. Test results, including BERA, are summarized in Table 5-8.

Of 140 patients, ENG was normal in 3.6 percent, was nonlocalizing in 17.1 percent, was suggestive of peripheral problems in 55.7 percent, and was suspicious of central pathology in 23.6 percent.

Comment

When the etiology of a SNHL was not confirmed by standard audiometric techniques or when the diagnosis was not known at the outset, BERA was accurate and reliable in determining the site of lesion, in ruling out acoustic tumor, as well as in confirming the degree of loss. Site-of-lesion capability was invaluable, particularly to the evaluation of unilateral impairment.

Once again, however, attempting to evaluate BERA results in cases of severe to profound loss proved nonlocalizing in several circumstances. Also, once again, these nonlocalizing data were included in that group representing instances in which BERA results were misleading clinically. In actuality, however, only four patients (21 percent) demonstrated abnormal findings that were clearly inconsistent with cochlear disease. Two patients exhibited abnormal wave V latencies, whereas another two patients exhibited abnormal central conductive times. In no case was wave V absent.

When this group was originally established, we anticipated a site-of-lesion dilemma in that we expected that a retrocochlear abnormality would clearly be responsible for approximately 25 percent of these cases of SNHL. The data generated were somewhat surprising. Evidently the test is unable to monitor discriminate effects of selective fiber depopulation of whatever etiology, which might well alter neural transmission to an extent to which SNHL is generated.[2] BERA, nonetheless, was accurate in determining no more than a cochlear site of lesion in 97.9 percent, which compares quite favorably again.

Group 5: Brain Stem Disorders

The diversity of this group, both in terms of clinical diagnosis and source of referral, demanded a departure from the format in which the preceding groups have been presented. Many of these cases were referred with a clinical diagnosis for BERA testing as confirmation. No universally common diagnostic protocol exists that would be presentable in this format. Each patient's presenting picture dictated an individualized diagnostic direction.

This group consists of 20 patients. Seventeen cases represent neurologically confirmed diagnoses of multiple sclerosis, whereas another three demonstrated examples of more unusual primary brain stem pathology. They are considered separately

Case 1

C.C. is a 16-year-old white male, originally evaluated by Vanderbilt University Medical Center and referred to The Otology Group by the Departments of Neurosurgery and Hearing and Speech Services. Sudden transient blindness with subsequent rapidly progressive decrements in auditory discrimination and ataxia presented in his evaluation. The CAT scan demonstrated a large intracranial mass in the region of the third ventricle. Pure tone and speech audiometry exhibited a moderate bilateral SNHL (Fig. 5-2). Upon presentation for BERA, the patient was lethargic, incoherent, and generally slept through the procedure. Results indicated normal formulation of wave I bilaterally, normal latency of wave III bilaterally, but a surprisingly large amplitude of wave III on the left. On the right, waves IV and V were abnormally separated and a left-sided wave V was not present (Fig. 5-3).

At surgery a large tumor was found to be extrinsically compressing the quadrigeminal plate, the anatomical localization of the interior colliculus. A clinical diagnosis of benign teratoma was later histopathologically established.

This case represents an example of the effects on brain stem auditory function by an extrinsic lesion. The resultant abnormal transmission is not only sensitively detected by BERA but also accurately localized.

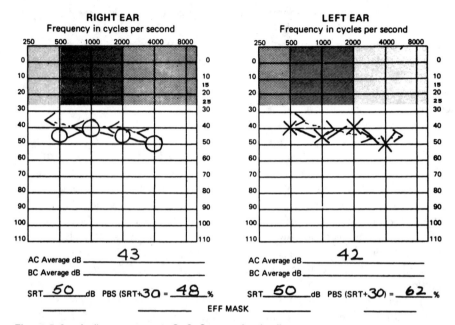

Figure 5–2. Audiogram, case 1, C. C. See text for details.

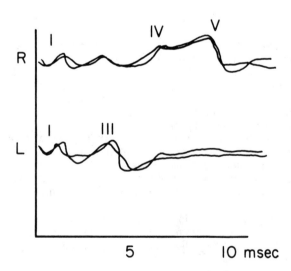

Figure 5-3. BERA, case 1, CC. See text for description. Anatomical localization of brain stem compression is accomplished with precision. (BERA procedural recording standards apply to this tracing as well as all subsequent recordings illustrated in this chapter; 0.1-msec click duration delivered at 40 to 60 dB SL re threshold unless otherwise indicated; repetition rate of eight per second; 50-Hz lower and 3000-Hz upper filters.

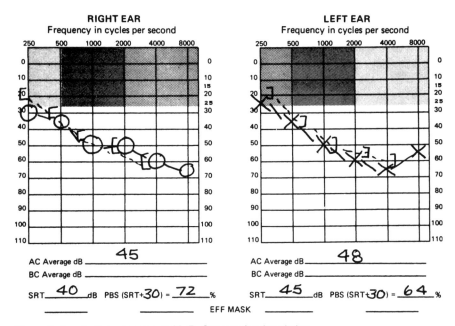

Figure 5–4. Audiogram, case 2, M. R. See text for description.

Case 2

M.R., a 56-year-old female, was evaluated by Vanderbilt University Neurology Clinic with a history of multiple cerebrovascular accidents (CVA) and a number of secondary clinical deficits. Further deterioration of long-standing hearing impairment, now with right hyperacusis and tinnitus, prompted referral for BERA. Audiometry is shown in Figure 5-4. BERA exhibits pro-

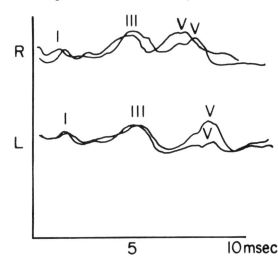

Figure 5-5. BERA, case 2, M. R. See text for description. Wave form abnormalities and test-retest variability is characteristic of brain stem dysfunction.

longation of wave III bilaterally with poor retest on right-sided stimulation (Fig. 5-5). Two weeks post-test she suffered a fatal myocardial infarction. At necropsy, multiple brain stem hemorrhages were identified, including an infarction in the caudal pontine tegmentum. Again, BERA's refinement of the concept of site lesion is clearly illustrated.

Case 3

B.L.S., a 4-year-old male, experienced progressive clumsiness, visual distrubances, and intermittent cephalgia. Evidence of marked personality changes over a 3-day period prompted hospital admission for evaluation.

Neurologic examination was consistent with a midbrain lesion. CAT scan outlined an enlarged third ventricle but no enhancing lesion. Audiometrics are shown in Figure 5-6. Acoustic reflexes were absent bilaterally with type A compliance curves; speech discrimination scores could not be obtained. BERA, obtained during sleep, elaborated repeatable but abnormal responses (Fig. 5-7). Wave I was identified bilaterally but was of unusually large amplitude. The second "bump" at the left is of unknown etiology. Binaural stimulation produced no change in wave I.

At craniotomy a large, unresectable intrinsic brain stem lesion was identified involving the anatomy up to the cochlear nuclei. A histological diagnosis of glioma (astrocytoma) was established. The child later expired. Autopsy was not performed.

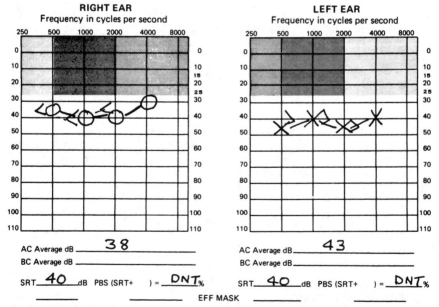

Figure 5–6. Audiogram, case 3, B.L.S. See text for details. Nondescript, flat, mild losses are characteristic of brain stem auditory dysfunction.

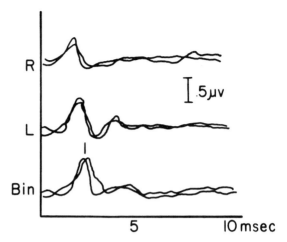

Figure 5-7. BERA, case 3, B. L. S. See text for description. Diffuse brain stem dysfunction is represented and multiple sclerosis is suggested. The remainder of the test battery clarified the diagnosis of tumor.

The remainder of this group was composed of 17 cases of multiple sclerosis that clinically involved brain stem pathways. All conformed to the general clinical portrait of multiple sclerosis, exhibiting clinical manifestations of multiple areas of demyelinization within the central nervous system. Symptomatic remission and exacerbation was a historical constant. Seven patients were referred by neurologists in an attempt to document brain stem pathology using the objectivity of BERA. Ten additional subjects presented for neurotologic work-up of a primary complaint of vertigo or loss of balance. As expected, a female predominance was exhibited (3 males; 14 females). Their ages ranges from 24 to 27 years (mean 36.3 years).

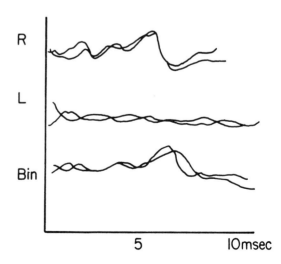

Figure 5-8. BERA, A. M. This 25-year-old female has neurologically defined multiple sclerosis. Note unilateral preservation of fairly normal wave form (right).

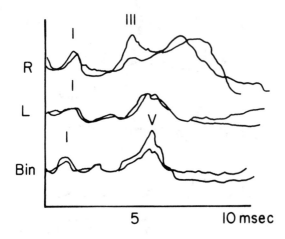

Figure 5-9. BERA, J. N. This 32-year-old male has multiple sclerosis. BERA findings are suggestive but not "classic."

Audiologically pure tone thresholds were normal for all frequencies in 14 subjects. One demonstrated a mild bilateral SNHL, whereas two others had mild to moderate, but symmetrical, high-frequency losses. All subjects elaborated speech discrimination scores better than 90 percent. Acoustic stapedial reflexes were elicited in 14 of these patients and showed no abnormal decay characteristics. An additional two subjects when tested failed to demonstrate reflexes bilaterally in the absence of middle ear pathology. A single patient was not tested using impedance techniques.

BERA in all 17 patients showed a variety of abnormal patterns. As we might well expect in a diffuse and commonly focal demyelinating process, these abnormalities exhibited no consistent pattern. Poor response reproduction on retest as well as poor summation on binaural stimulation were frequently noted. Wave I was identified on one or both sides in 14 subjects,

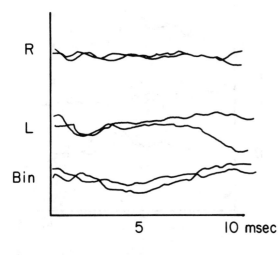

Figure 5-10. BERA, N. F. This 44-year-old female has multiple sclerosis and was very symptomatic at the time of testing. This tracing represents an extreme in wave form breakdown and dysynchrony.

whereas being represented bilaterally normal in 10. Only one of the 17 exhibited a normal wave V, this being identified only unilaterally. Figures 5-8 to 5-10 represent the range of abnormalities demonstrated by these 17 subjects.

Comment

These cases clearly illustrate that BERA can be useful in demonstrating primary or extrinsic brain stem pathology, as it reflects brain stem auditory pathway dysfunction. In the absence of any definitive, noninvasive evaluation of the status of the brain stem, both the objectivity and sensitivity of BERA heralds it as a primary addition to the physician's armamentarium available to document an often-elusive clinical diagnosis. This is particularly true when considering demyelinating processes, specifically multiple sclerosis.

The patient presenting to the otoneurosurgeon with some form of balance disturbance must clearly have multiple sclerosis added to a differential diagnosis including acoustic tumor, non-Meniere's vertigo, and so forth. In conjunction with the appropriate clinical picture, BERA findings of bilateral dysynchrony, poor test-retest reliability, and insufficient amplitude simulation on binaural stimulation all strongly suggest brain stem involvement. The capability exists not only to confirm a clinically insecure diagnosis but also to accurately localize within the brain stem neuroanatomy the "site of lesion ." Starr and Achor[4] as well as Nodar[12] have clearly defined the clinical ability of BERA in this context.

Brain stem auditory responses also have been shown to vary with the stage of process of multiple sclerosis as it exists in the exacerbation-remission continuum. Possible usefulness in follow-up and perhaps in predicting exacerbation have immense therapeutic implications. These suggestions rely heavily upon the sensitivity of BERA, which is nicely exhibited in the evaluation of one of our patients who is willing to be retested once or twice a week. This female subject reports frequent episodes of the disease often achieving crisis proportions interspersed by brief periods of remission. Diagnosed 1 year ago, she has been tested now 18 times in the last 5 months. When she reports feeling well, BERA will exhibit variations from minor effects to higher levels (wave V) to complete normality, seen on only three occasions. At her clinical worst (four test occasions), no response is noted bilaterally. The intermediate 11 sessions all yielded a wave I and a wave III form. Binaural summation is only variably identified.

The abnormally large amplitudes of wave I commonly seen in these instances of brain stem pathology are also occasionally seen in the other early wave forms. This phenomenon has been observed by other clinicians,[13,14] but remains unexplained physiologically.

It is important to restate a point presented in the preceding chapter relative to the capability of BERA in establishing a diagnosis. An absent or delayed wave V does not always necessarily relate a diagnosis of acoustic tumor. Abnormal BERA data suggests a wide variety of pathological processes, the differential diagnosis of which depends largely upon the remainder of the test battery for elucidation. BERA, alone, is simply not able to suggest a histopathological correlate to its abnormal response.

BERA, nevertheless, presents itself as possibly one of a few noninvasive objective evaluators of the status of the brain stem in the question of primary pathology. Its usefulness in the early diagnosis of an as yet neurologically unconfirmed pathology is suggested but still remains to be evaluated.

Group 6: Confirmation of Threshold

This group is composed of those individuals who either could not or would not cooperate with standard audiometric formats sufficiently enough to be able to generate an audiogram. In this regard, they represented behavioral failures. Ten patients (5 females and 5 males) and 20 ears were evaluated. They ranged in age from 2 months to 52 years, with a mean of 12.3 years. For the eight testable patients, average pure tone averages or voluntary threshold was 50.2 dB. The patients generally underwent no special testing within the neurotologic scheme.

Audiological confirmation of BERA results was obviously difficult to achieve. Two children, untestable by traditional techniques, were consistent after three subsequent repeated observations of function, with a degree of peripheral loss indicated by BERA. For the remaining eight patients there was (at least) good audiological indication of invalid threshold responses on routine testing. Poor retest reliability was most commonly encountered. In these cases otological examination and impedance audiometry supported BERA findings. In all eight at least one audiological evaluation was acknowledged as possibly invalid. An additional two patients, after repeated attempts at behavioral testing, eventually produced repeatable data consistent with BERA thresholds. In another eight ears, BERA was found to indicate a high-frequency peripheral loss significantly better than that elaborated by initial behavioral testing.

In one infant and one severely retarded child, some objective insight into the capability of the peripheral auditory system was sought. Thresholds were obtained in approximately 1 hour. They, however, remain unconfirmed.

Comment

Very early in this chapter we acknowledged that the site-of-lesion surgical emphasis of the clinical practice within the Otology Group did not find confirmation of threshold to constitute a major portion of BERA's usefulness. In many otology and otolaryngology practices, particularly those in which a high percentage of the patient population is pediatric, BERA would make a more significant contribution.

Often the information generated is more specific and reliable than that obtained over a time period of two to three times longer using traditional methods. This well-established fact, nonetheless, does not preclude the contribution of these techniques, notably behavioral and impedance audiometry. BERA, one must remember, generates information regarding neurophysiological auditory thresholds as they reflect the integrity of the peripheral mechanisms and the more central brain stem auditory projections. The technique excludes evaluation of the cortical integrative aspects that actually define "hearing" as that perception and interpretation of sound energy. This cortical integrative function is only evaluated by traditional behavioral and, by definition, subjective formats. Only speech audiometry can evaluate what a patient "hears."

Our limited experience in this category allows us to present BERA as effective reinforcement of behavioral failures. Presented as a part of a battery of tests including impedance and behavioral audiometry (and occasionally E Co G), BERA allows for an effective screening device in high-risk patients (neonates).[15] The test's objectivity defines its implied role in the therapeutic area of rehabilitation, be it psychiatric or auditory.

Group 7: Miscellaneous

Thirty-seven patients (53 pathological) ears exhibited pathology not classifiable in any one of the preceding categories. Most prominent disease entities of this group included facial nerve lesions, tinnitus, and von Recklinghausen's disease. In addition, there was a single arterio-venous malformation, a single central nervous system disorder with unconfirmed brain stem pathology, and one case in which posterior fossa myelography was misleading. The mean age of this population was 33.7 years, with 28 females and 27 male ears represented.

Pure tone averages ranged from 0 to 42 dB with a mean of 24.2 dB. Mean PB function was 92.4 percent. Test results, including BERA, are summarized in Table 5–9.

ENG suggested peripheral disease in 35 percent, central pathology in

TABLE 5–9.

	BERA	IRD	PPX	CT	PFM
N:	53	37	49	43	20
Normal retrocochlear apparatus suggested	94.3%	89.2%	87.8%	97.7%	95.0%
Retrocochlear pathology suggested	5.7%	10.8%	12.2%	2.3%	5.0%

20 percent, and was normal in 40 percent of the 20 subjects tested. Nonlocalizing data appeared in 50 percent.

Comment

BERA was positive in three patients, in each of whom the study suggested brain stem pathology. One of these patients had a normal neurological evaluation; another represented an abnormality opposite a large cholesteatoma secondary to which brain stem shift was suspected; and the last case exhibited a large temporoparietal arterio-venous malformation confirmed angiographically.

The abnormal CAT scan reported was elaborated by the large cholesteatoma indirectly diagnosed as a result of its ventricle shifting effect.

A single symptomatic patient (unsteadiness) demonstrated abnormal plain petrous pyramid x-rays, and a pantopaque posterior fossa study failed to fill the suspect internal auditory canal. No filling defect or mass effect was however suggested. BERA and other studies were unremarkable. We suggested close follow-up and repeat studies in 6 months to 1 year. The very anxious patient, however, strongly favored the alternative of exploration. Subsequent middle fossa exposure of the internal auditory canal, preserving hearing, confirmed the normal findings suggested by BERA.

SUMMARY

Commonly referred to as "the wave of the future," BERA, based on continued clinical verification, is firmly established as "the wave of the present." Its sensitivity and accuracy within its totally objective context make BERA a very practical inclusion into the neurotologist's clinical armamentarium. The expansion of the concept of "retrocochlear" into eighth nerve and brain stem confirms the utility of BERA in the site-of-lesion protocol. Its objectivity and accuracy similarly propose BERA as very effective support for behavioral and traditional format failures within the field of threshold determination. Certain limitations, however, restrict the application, in all circumstances, of this sophisticated test to operation within the context of a battery of tests, its role being entirely adjunctive.

Although remarkably useful operating within its present constraints, the future of BERA suggests unlimited utility. Increased and more detailed understanding of the neurophysiology of the auditory system, elaborated largely by BERA, suggest even greater possible contributions to the evaluation of the neurotologically impaired. An increased understanding of central auditory dysfunction and intrinsic abnormality of neural transmission alone suggest major advancements potentially created through the technology of electric response audiometry.

There is little question that BERA represents a major contribution to neurotological diagnosis. Its incorporation into contemporary neuroaudiology is strongly suggested.

REFERENCES

1. Selters, W. A., Brackmann, D. E.: Acoustic tumor detection with brainstem electric response audiometry. Arch Otolaryngol 103:181-187, 1977.
2. Glasscock, M. E., Jackson, C. G., Josey, A. F., Dickens, J. R. E., and Weit, R. J.: Brainstem evoked response audiometry in a clinical practice. Laryngoscope 89:1021-1034, 1979.
3. Starr, A., and Hamilton, A. E.: Correlation between confirmed sites of neurological lesions and abnormalities of far field auditory brainstem responses. Electroencephalogr Clin Neurophysiol 41:595-608, 1976.
4. Starr, A., and Achor, L. I.: Auditory brainstem responses in neurologic disease. Arch Neurol 32:761-768, 1975.
5. Stockard, J. T., and Rossiter, V. S.: Clinical and pathologic correlates of brainstem auditory response abnormalities. Neurology 27:316-325, 1977.
6. Hecox, K., and Galambos, R.: Brainstem auditory evoked responses in human infants and adults. Arch Otolaryngol 99:30-33, 1974.
7. Jerger, J., Mouldin, L., and Anthony, I: Brainstem evoked response audiometry. Audio-Hear Edu 4:17-24, 1978.
8. Berlin, C. I., and Dobie, R. A.: Electrophysiologic measures of auditory function via electroencephalograph and brainstem evoked response. In Rintelmann, W. F. (ed.), Hearing Assessment. Baltimore, University Park Press, 1978.
9. Josey, A. F., Jackson, C. G., and Glasscock, M. E.: Brainstem evoked response audiometry in confirmed eighth nerve tumors. Am J Otolaryngol 1:285-290, 1980.
10. Witten, R., and Wade, C. T.: Computed tomography in acoustic tumor diagnosis. Acoustic Tumors, Vol. I: Diagnosis, House, W. F., and Luetje, C. M. (eds.), pp. 253-277. Baltimore, University Park Press, 1979.
11. Committee on Hearing and Equilibrium of the American Academy of Opthalmology and Otolaryngology: Trans Am Acad Ophthalmol Otolaryngol 76:1462, 1972.
12. Nodar, R. H., Hahn, J. Jr., and Levine, H. L.: Brainstem auditory evoked potentials in determining site of lesion of brainstem gliomas in children. Laryngoscope 90:358-265, 1980.
13. Coats, A. C., and Martin, J. L.: Human auditory nerve action potentials and brainstem evoked responses. Arch Otolaryngol 103:605-622, 1977.
14. Nodar, R. H.: Personal communication.
15. Schulman-Galambos, C., and Galambos, R.: Brainstem evoked response audiometry in newborn hearing screening. Arch Otolaryngol 105:86-90, 1979.

INDEX

125